....

Radiation Injury

Frontiers of Radiation Therapy and Oncology

Vol. 32

Series Editors   *John L. Meyer*, San Francisco, Calif.
                  Jerome M. Vaeth, San Francisco, Calif.

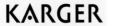

Basel · Freiburg · Paris · London · New York ·
New Delhi · Bangkok · Singapore · Tokyo · Sydney

32nd San Francisco Cancer Symposium, San Francisco, Calif.

....

Radiation Injury

Advances in Management and Prevention

Volume Editor   *John L. Meyer*, San Francisco, Calif.

59 figures, and 29 tables, 1999

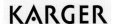

Basel · Freiburg · Paris · London · New York ·
New Delhi · Bangkok · Singapore · Tokyo · Sydney

Frontiers of Radiation Therapy and Oncology
....
John L. Meyer

Director, Department of Radiation Oncology
Saint Francis Memorial Hospital
900 Hyde Street
San Francisco, CA 94109 (USA)

Library of Congress Cataloging-in-Publication Data
San Francisco Cancer Symposium (32nd:1997)
Radiation injury / 32nd San Francisco Cancer Symposium, San Francisco, Calif., March 1–2, 1997;
volume editor, John L. Meyer.
(Frontiers of radiation therapy and oncology; vol. 32)
Includes bibliographical references and index.
1. Cancer – Radiotherapy – Complications Congresses.   2. Radiation injuries Congresses.
I. Meyer, John, 1949–   . II. Title.   III. Series.
[DNLM: 1. Radiation Injuries Congresses.   2. Radiotherapy – adverse effects Congresses.
W3 FR935 v.32 1999]
RC271.R3S3 1997
616.99′40642–dc21
ISBN 3–8055–6802–9

Bibliographic Indices. This publication is listed in bibliographic services, including Current Contents® and Index Medicus.

Drug Dosage. The authors and the publisher have exerted every effort to ensure that drug selection and dosage set forth in this text are in accord with current recommendations and practice at the time of publication. However, in view of ongoing research, changes in government regulations, and the constant flow of information relating to drug therapy and drug reactions, the reader is urged to check the package insert for each drug for any change in indications and dosage and for added warnings and precautions. This is particularly important when the recommended agent is a new and/or infrequently employed drug.

All rights reserved. No part of this publication may be translated into other languages, reproduced or utilized in any form or by any means electronic or mechanical, including photocopying, recording, microcopying, or by any information storage and retrieval system, without permission in writing from the publisher.

© Copyright 1999 by S. Karger AG, P.O. Box, CH–4009 Basel (Switzerland)
Printed in Switzerland on acid-free paper by Reinhardt Druck, Basel
ISBN 3–8055–6802–9

Contents

....

In Memoriam

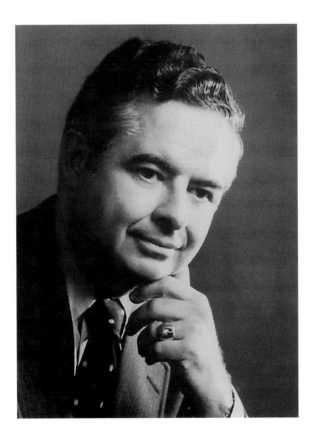

The end of 1998 was marked by the passing of Dr. Jerome Vaeth, who founded the San Francisco Cancer Symposium and its proceedings, this Frontiers book series. His energies invigorated the two over the next 25 years, creating and continuing a world forum recognized for the discussion of issues important to cancer care.

Dr. Vaeth contributed to the field of oncology in many ways. Born in Colorado, he studied medicine and received his medical degree from Saint Louis University in 1950. In 1952, he applied for training in therapeutic radiology at the Penrose Cancer Hospital in his native Colorado Springs, under the Leadership of Dr. Juan del Regato. As his teacher later observed, 'Vaeth was among the earliest of a young generation of physicians who understood the challenge of the new discipline. He was a model resident, enthralled by the protean variety of malignant tumors, the intricacies and limitations of their morphologic diagnoses, and invigorated by his increasing clinical experience.' In 1956, Dr. Vaeth was certified by the American Board of Radiology. That year, only six other candidates were certified in therapeutic radiology by the Board. Following completion of his training, Dr. Vaeth was awarded a fellowship by the American Cancer Society to spend an additional year at the Curie Foundation of Paris and at the Holt Radium Institute of Manchester.

Upon his return to the United States, he took a position as Assistant Professor of Radiology at the University of California in San Francisco. He was to assist the recently appointed Professor Franz Buschke, and as his assistant Dr. Vaeth created one of the first residency training programs in radiation oncology. In the 1960's, the Mount Zion Hospital of San Francisco sought to create a center distinguished for the treatment of cancer. Dr. Buschke recommended his trusted assistant. Thus, Dr. Vaeth became director of the Claire Zellerbach Saroni Memorial Tumor Institute.

In 1972, he became the director of radiotherapy services for a consortium of San Francisco hospitals, the West Coast Cancer Foundation, and established his offices at the St. Mary's Hospital and Medical Center. As director of a multi-hospital residency program, he continued to dedicate himself to the training of radiation oncologists. He created the San Francisco Cancer Symposium, carefully prepared and conducted with wide participation and attendance, and he edited the proceedings of these conferences, which have been published annually as this Frontiers series.

These publications, with their far-ranging scientific explorations, have been just one mark of his fortitude and dedication. We celebrate his spirit of investigation and leadership in oncology, and know that his influence in radiotherapy will be felt for many years to come.

John Meyer, MD

Foreword

In the clinic, observed reactions to radiotherapy range from minor to serious, and from transient to permanent. It is a remarkable part of our experience that the most serious radiation injuries are often the last to be apparent: late reactions in spinal cord, brain, bone and other organs that may be devastating and permanent, and may have no early signs. Physician concern for these debilitating effects permeates the clinical practice of radiation, and influences the selection of treatments on a day-to-day basis. Optimal utilization of radiation as a cancer therapy requires a clear understanding of the range of the major tissue sequelae that can occur, including their risk of occurrence, natural history and treatment. This understanding leads to better clinical practice: greater confidence in recommending aggressive radiation treatment programs when appropriate, or the selection of other therapies when they are safer and equally effective.

In our current world of multimodality therapy, it is especially important to understand new risk factors for radiation sequelae, especially the interactions of external radiotherapy with many new treatment methods – systemic cytotoxic and biologic agents, and recent innovations in surgery, brachytherapy, and radiosurgery. Dose escalation with conformal radiotherapy alone may introduce new or previously unrecognized radiation sequelae. An understanding of these effects is required as the basis for development of new strategies to prevent injury from radiotherapy delivery.

When clinically significant problems develop following radiotherapy, are they actually a result of the radiotherapy? It is essential to understand the other clinical possibilities that exist in the differential diagnosis. These other possibilities often include consideration for tumor progression, adverse chemotherapy effects, secondary infections or paraneoplastic responses. Our understanding of radiation sequelae must be matched by an equally accurate understanding of these alternative possibilities, and the methods to diagnose and modify them.

Minor radiation reactions during therapy, the inflammatory reactions that occur as part of the normal tissue responses to radiotherapy, may be an expected part of therapy. But they also may be quite debilitating to the patient during the treatment course. Their frequency and occasional severity warrant discussion of their successful management, including ways to facilitate a more comfortable therapy course for the patient.

Once a major radiation injury has occurred, we must be knowledgeable about the methods to improve its outcome. A range of treatment possibilities usually exist, including initial drug therapies, minor surgical treatments or other conservative methods. Earlier intervention may reduce the compounding effect of the developing clinical problems, one leading to another. It is also important to understand the indications and outcomes of more aggressive managements, such as surgical organ diversions or major tissue resections, so that reasonable judgement may be in the patient's favor.

Clinically significant sequelae after radiotherapy should be uncommon, but do occur with a small incidence even after expert inital therapy. When they develop, it is important to have resource information about their management. It is also important to review all possible causes of them, for prevention in subsequent cases. This volume brings together an outstanding faculty for the discussion of the most modern strategies in the prevention and treatment of radiation injury.

John Meyer, MD, San Francisco

Meyer JL (ed): Radiation Injury. Advances in Management and Prevention.
Front Radiat Ther Oncol. Basel, Karger, 1999, vol 32, pp 1–8

....

Radiation Effects on Normal Tissues

H. Rodney Withers, William H. McBride

Roy E. Coats Research Laboratories, Department of Radiation Oncology and
Jonsson Comprehensive Cancer Center, University of California,
Los Angeles, Calif., USA

The underlying theme of this introductory paper is to outline briefly the changes in our understanding of normal tissue responses which have crept in quietly, like the San Francisco fog, during the more than 25 years since the first symposium in this series on normal tissues.

Pathobiology of Tissue Responses

There are three generic types of normal tissue responses to radiation based on the kinetics of their development: acute, late and consequential. Acute effects develop during a standard 6- or 7-week course of radiation therapy and can be modified by altering the intensity of treatment. Late effects develop weeks, months or years after the end of treatment and the only basis for modifying their severity by altering treatment fractionation patterns is on the statistics of prior experience. Consequential late effects are only seen in tissues underlying an epithelial surface, and their incidence and severity track the severity of the acute response, e.g. of oropharyngeal or rectal mucosa. In general, they appear earlier than standard late effects.

The kinetics of the radiation response depend upon the turnover kinetics of the tissue, determined by the rate of cell renewal and the lifetime of differentiating progeny. For example, thrombocytopenia and leukopenia develop early whereas anemia develops slowly, reflecting the slow turnover of differentiating and differentiated erythrocytes compared with the fast turnover of platelets and leukocytes. Late responses are therefore thought to reflect a slow turnover of putative target cells in tissues, e.g. oligodendrocytes in brain and spinal cord, fibroblasts in the dermis, tubule epithelium in the kidney.

Vascular Injury

Vascular injury is a late effect which is poorly understood. Sometimes it is apparently an endothelial response as in the Budd-Chiari syndrome following irradiation of the liver, whereas in other situations the subintima and muscle wall of the vasculature degenerate [1]. The former appears earlier than the latter. Vascular injury can presumably add to the severity of other late injuries, but there is little evidence for its having a primary causal role except in radiation hepatitis in man and in some, but not all animals [1].

Response as a Function of Dose per Fraction

Early responses to multiple, clinically relevant dose fractions (e.g. 1–3 Gy) are only slightly dependent upon fraction size. By contrast, the severity of late responses increases strongly with increase in dose per fraction. This can be explained by a relatively greater proportion of the injury to acutely responding tissues being due to single-hit (α-type) injury which is not repairable and hence not dependent upon fraction size. By contrast, late responding tissues are relatively more susceptible to interactive (β-type) ionization lesions and hence become increasingly more damaged as the dose is increased. Conversely, they are proportionally more spared by reducing the dose per fraction. In terms of the coefficients for single-hit (α) and multi-hit (β) injury, the late responding tissues have a low α/β ratio. This ratio is high for consequential late responses, resembling in this way the fractionation responses of acutely responding tissues [2].

Regeneration

Repopulation by surviving cells in all steady-state normal tissues is preceded by a lag time after the start of a course of radiation therapy, reflecting the time required for homeostatic mechanisms to respond to the developing injury. The essential cellular regeneration response triggered by injury is a change in the cell-loss pattern. In steady state, one mitotic division produces, on average, one stem cell and one differentiating cell. To regenerate itself, the tissue must restore its stock of stem cells by reducing the cell loss rate from 1.0 per mitotic division. Some tissues reduce it to 0 (e.g. jejunal crypts) and regenerate quickly, others (e.g. skin) may only reduce it to about 0.5 and regenerate less quickly. The seminiferous epithelium shows little change and mostly continues in a steady state, producing sperm in numbers reduced in direct proportion to the depletion of stem cells.

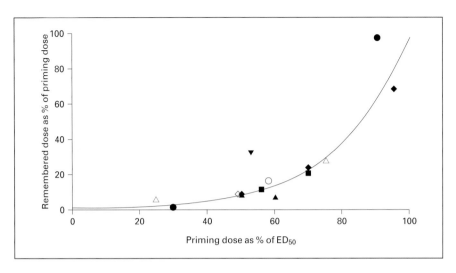

Fig. 1. The data show the effect of a prior dose of irradiation on the ED_{50} for myelitis in various experimental animals [3]. The ordinate shows the reduction in ED_{50} for a second course of irradiation, as a percentage of the dose given in the first course, that is the percentage 'remembered' dose. The abscissa plots the size of the first treatment as a percentage of the ED_{50} for a single course. The higher the dose in the first regimen, the greater the 'remembered' dose, once doses above about 50% of the ED_{50} are given. [Reprinted with permission Pergamon Press.]

Remembered Dose

Acutely responding normal tissues regenerate themselves quickly, and provided their stem cell population is not excessively depleted, can soon 'forget' they had been injured. In general, after an acutely responding tissue has fully regenerated itself to an essentially normal state, its response to a second treatment is similar to that from the initial treatment.

It now appears that the same principle applies to late responding tissues. But, because there are long lag times before injury begins to manifest itself in slowly responding tissues, there are also long delays before their surviving 'target' clonogenic cells are stimulated to regenerate. Thus, late responding tissues are slower to return to a normal fully restored status, and hence to 'forget' their prior injury.

Therefore, the safety with which a late responding tissue can be re-irradiated depends upon the size of first dose (i.e. the severity of injury) (fig. 1), and upon the elapsed time (i.e. the extent of regeneration) after the first treatment. Figure 1 shows the extent of residual injury in irradiated spinal cords as a function of the severity of prior radiation injury, when the second course of treatment is delayed for times long enough to allow maximal recovery [3]. This ability of late responding tissues to tolerate re-irradiation was not appreciated in past times when late injury was considered to result from vascular injury.

Tolerance Doses and Functional Subunits

Although the kidney is a large organ, containing large numbers of cells, it does not tolerate irradiation well. The radiosensitivity of its tubule cells is similar to that for epithelial cells of skin or intestinal mucosa. The low 'tolerance' dose reflects the structural packaging of cells into small functional subunits (nephrons). If all nephrons contained 10^4 clonogenic tubule cells, then a dose that reduced cell survival to 10^{-4} would leave, on average, only one cell per nephron. Because of the random nature of cell killing by radiation, about 37% of the nephrons would have zero cells surviving, the others containing one or, occasionally, a few cells. Thus, a relatively low dose is very damaging, and furthermore, the damage would increase rapidly with relatively small increments in dose. Clearly, if the nephrons each contained 10^8 cells, the tolerance dose would be doubled. The tolerance of organs can depend strongly upon the architecture of its functional and structural subunits.

The higher tolerance of other tissues, e.g. skin epithelium, can be understood in terms of the mobility of its clonogenic cells through their not being structurally confined. A surviving clonogenic cell in skin can repopulate, even during radiation therapy, to cover several mm^2, and with time, can form quite large islands of epithelium in an otherwise ulcerated area. Thus, in operational terms, its functional subunit is large.

Volume Effects and Tolerance

The decreased tolerance associated with an increase in treatment volume does not reflect an increase in radiation cytotoxicity. It may reflect a decreased ability of a large area of severe injury to heal, or of the patient to tolerate a large area of injury, or it may reflect loss of functional reserve (e.g. of lungs, liver, parotid). It may also reflect the increased heterogeneity in dose distribution in a large volume, resulting in some areas getting high total doses given in proportionately large doses per fraction, creating an illusion that the increased injury was due to the large volume per se. Or in some organs in which functional subunits are arranged in series, e.g. spinal cord, it may reflect a higher probability that one functional subunit will be sterilized, resulting in a broken link in a chain: the more 'links' exposed, the higher the probability that one will fail, resulting in expression of injury of the organ as a whole.

Genetic Variability

Norman et al. [4] first drew attention to the fact that if a small proportion of the population was more radiosensitive than the majority, then the 'tolerance' doses used in radiation therapy are generally too low. The best known cause of increased radiosensitivity is a mutation of the ataxia telangiectasia gene. While homozygous A-T gene mutants are rare, heterozygotes could make up 2–5% of the population. Although heterozygote radiosensitivity has been shown to be quite variable, it is not greatly different from normal (non-A-T mutant gene carriers). Nevertheless, fractionation of dose can amplify small differences per fraction into quite large ultimate differences in cell depletion, and it remains to be determined whether tolerance doses are unduly influenced by a slightly more radiosensitive subpopulation of people. This possibility would be greater if it were also true that A-T heterozygotes are more likely than average to develop cancer, increasing thereby their representation within a population of patients receiving radiation therapy.

Apoptosis

Radiation can cause cells to die by apoptosis, as well as by a disruption of their reproductive integrity at mitosis. Apoptotic death is associated with interphase (nonmitotic) death, e.g. in lymphocytes, serous cells in the parotid, and a proportion of cells in most epithelia, but it can also occur in cycling cells at different phases of the cell cycle, including after mitosis. Since it has always existed, its recognition as a form of cell death does not change its role in tissue responses to irradiation. However, it is a process that can be augmented and suppressed, e.g. by mutation or altered expression of genes such as p53, abl, bc12 family, myc that are involved in carcinogenesis. This gives hope that the process may be exploitable in attempts to modify the therapeutic ratio.

Wound Healing

Radiation can reduce wound tensile strength but only after high doses, and the weakness usually persists for only a limited period of time. There is, however, a small window of time after surgery or other physical trauma when relatively small doses can restrain wound healing and, more importantly, prevent the hyperplastic responses seen in keloid formation, pterygia and, perhaps myointimal hyperplasia in blood vessels after angioplasty. The timing of the maximal effectiveness of radiation coincides with times when radiation injury could inhibit the contractile phase of wound healing mediated by myofibroblasts. However, the mechanism by which small doses inhibit exuberant hyperplastic responses is still unknown.

Pneumonitis Outside the Radiation Field

A proportion of patients receiving lung irradiation appear to develop pneumonitis beyond that portion of the lungs actually within the radiation field. This is most likely due to extension of the inflammatory response outside the irradiated area and mediated by upregulation of cell adhesion molecules that allow cells to extravasate into the surrounding tissue. It may be exacerbated by infection, but there is evidence that in some circumstances autoimmune-like reactions are possible, that may be genetically determined [5].

Cytokine Induction

An early effect of irradiation, occurring within hours, is to reorchestrate cellular gene expression [6–10]. There is little evidence, as yet, for induction of classic DNA repair enzymes after exposure. Rather, inflammatory molecules such as cytokines (e.g. IL-1, TNF-α, interferon, etc.), proteases (e.g. plasminogen activator), cell adhesion molecules (e.g. ICAM-1, selectins) and eicosanoids (prostaglandins, thromboxanes, leukotrienes) predominate to form a well-coordinated response to tissue injury. With time after irradiation, there are subsequent 'waves' of gene expression, perpetrated mainly by cell loss, that extend as long as injury persists and that represent attempts at tissue regeneration, that may be eventually abortive. The 'lag time' that precedes expression of tissue failure in late effects tissues is therefore a time of ongoing molecular and cellular responses. The consequences of this induced gene expression in terms of the radiation response of the tissue (and tumor) still have to be fully explored. Many of the prodromal effects of irradiation that can not be attributed to cell loss, such as acute vascular leak and edema, hyper- and hypotension, fatigue, are probably due to production of cytokines while growth factors involved in tissue regeneration will precipitate the 'avalanche' effect seen in late effect tissues, where the time to failure is more dose-dependent than it is in acute effects tissues. Recognition of the molecular and cellular processes underlying the tissue response are important in that they provide a target for therapy in attempts to ameliorate normal tissue reactions and tumor radiosensitivity. They might also provide a basis for genetic variation between individual responses to radiotherapy.

Fatigue

An important side effect of radiation therapy which has received remarkably little attention is the fatigability which is generally greater the greater the treatment volume. It is common in patients receiving total body irradiation and is also a feature of much chemotherapy.

While the mechanism is not known, similar side effects are seen with biologic treatments (e.g. interferon, IL-1, TNF-α). Since these cytokines are produced following irradiation, it is possible that they could be released in sufficient quantity to induce fatigability, especially when large volumes of tissue are irradiated. Another possible source of cytokines that may contribute to general fatigue is the tumor itself.

Postradiation Recovery

Contrary to previous concepts, it now appears that some radiation injury may be modulated by postirradiation treatment [10–12]. Given the nature of the radiation-induced inflammatory response noted earlier, it is not surprising that there are numerous studies on the effects of steroids and NSAIDs on radiation responses. Although there are conflicting reports, taken collectively, the experience is that both can exert beneficial therapeutic influence. Steroids most commonly delay rather than prevent late reactions, but do affect early responses related to vascular leak and there is a need for more studies with measurable molecular endpoints to determine the effectiveness of these agents.

Angiotensin-converting enzyme (ACE) inhibitors, such as captopril – a free-thiol compound used to reduce vascular resistance in patients with hypertension, heart failure, or chronic renal disease – are effective in the prophylaxis of radiation pneumonitis and nephropathy in rats. The beneficial effects of such inhibitors are thought to be mediated by their systemic and renal hemodynamic effects through the vasculature. Other vasoactive agents such as pentoxifylline have also been shown to modify late radiation responses, especially in soft tissues. This drug can alter red cell deformability, but has many other effects including blocking TNF production and affecting G_2M arrest, which make it hard to determine its major mechanism of radioprotection.

Clearly modification of late tissue responses to irradiation are an area of fruitful future research and will be a topic for further discussion during this meeting.

Acknowledgment

Supported by PHS grant No. CA-31612 awarded by the National Cancer Institute, DHHS.

References

1   Withers HR, Peters LJ, Kogelnik HD: The pathobiology of late effects of irradiation; in Meyn RE, Withers HR (eds): Radiation Biology in Cancer Research. New York, Raven Press, 1980, pp 439–448.
2   Withers HR, Peters LJ, Taylor JMG et al: Late normal tissue sequelae from radiation therapy for carcinoma of the tonsil: Patterns of fractionation study of radiobiology. Int J Radiat Oncol Biol Phys 1995;33:563–568.
3   Mason KA, Withers HR, Chiang CS: Late effects of radiation on the lumbar spinal cord of guinea pigs: Re-treatment tolerance. Int J Radiat Oncol Biol Phys 1993;26:643–648.
4   Norman A, Kagan AR, Chan SL: The importance of genetics for the optimization of radiation therapy. A hypothesis. Am J Clin Oncol 1988;11:84–88.
5   McBride WH, Vegesna VJ: Role of the thymus in radiation-induced lung damage after bone marrow transplantation. Radiat Res 1997;147:501–505.
6   Hong JH, Chiang CS, Campbell IL, Sun JR, Withers HR, McBride WH: Induction of acute phase gene expression by brain irradiation. Int J Radiat Oncol Biol Phys 1995;33:619–626.
7   McBride WH: Cytokine cascades in late normal tissue radiation responses (editorial). Int J Radiat Oncol Biol Phys 1995;33:233–234.
8   McBride WH, Chiang CS, Hong JH, Withers HR: Molecular and cellular responses of the brain to radiotherapy; in Khayat D, Hortobagyi G (eds): Current Clinical Topics in Cancer Chemotherapy. Cambridge, Blackwell Science, 1997.
9   Michalowski A: On radiation damage to normal tissues and its treatment. Acta Oncol 1990;29: 1017–1023.
10   Michalowski A: On radiation damage to normal tissues and its treatment. II. Anti-inflammatory drugs. Acta Oncol 1994;33:139–157.
11   Hopewell JW: Modifying Radiation Injury to Normal Tissues: New Opportunities. Front Radiat Ther Oncol. Basel, Karger, 1999, pp 9–20.
12   Ward WF, Molteni A, Ts'ao C-H: Radiation-induced endothelial dysfunction and fibrosis in rat lung: Modification by the angiotensin-coverting enzyme inhibitor CL242817. Radiat Res 1989;117: 342–350.

Dr. H.R. Withers, Department of Radiation Oncology, UCLA Medical Center, 10833 LeConte Avenue, Los Angeles, CA 90095-1714 (USA)

Meyer JL (ed): Radiation Injury. Advances in Management and Prevention.
Front Radiat Ther Oncol. Basel, Karger, 1999, vol 32, pp 9–20

....

Modifying Radiation Injury to Normal Tissues: New Opportunities

J.W. Hopewell

Normal Tissue Radiobiology Group, Research Institute (University of Oxford),
The Churchill Hospital, Oxford, UK

Introduction

To improve the therapeutic ratio in radiotherapy the conventional approach has been to consider ways of enhancing tumour response without adversely affecting normal tissue morbidity. Several approaches have been tried including the modification of radiotherapy dose fractionation schedules and attempts to sensitize hypoxic cells in solid tumours to radiation. While limited success has been reported [1], the results obtained with the latter approach have not been achieved without concerns about the toxicity of some of the agents used.

An alternative and exciting approach that is now attracting considerable interest is the possibilities for modifying the expression of normal tissue injury. Normal tissue reactions might be modified by intervention prior to radiotherapy, at the time of radiation treatment (radioprotection) or after irradiation has been completed (modulation). Classical radioprotectors act by enhancing the repair of irradiation-induced sublethal injury, thus increasing clonogenic cell survival. These agents, by definition, are not selective for normal tissues and although again they have achieved some limited success, their use has also been hampered by toxicity [2]. Intervention after radiotherapy has been targeted to be selective for normal tissues. Agents previously used in the clinical management of a range of diseases, not related to radiation exposure, have been used. Many were already known to have minimal toxicity when administered over long periods. Two general approaches have been proposed: (1) to intervene prior to the development of damage in order to ameliorate the expression of damage (prophylaxis), and (2) to reduce the severity of established radiation-induced injury (treatment). Evidence for the validity of such approaches will be reviewed. Factors associated with their introduction into clinical studies will be discussed in relation to the requirement to improve the therapeutic ratio.

Modulation of Normal Tissue Injury

Prophylaxis

There is considerable interest in the potential use of growth factors for the modulation of acute reactions in normal tissues. The haematopoietic system is the most studied tissue, in relation to growth regulation of its constituent cell lineages. After cytotoxic insult, granulocytopenia is usually the most important deficit. Normally recovery would be slow, leading to the onset of secondary and tertiary adverse events. The use of exogenous granulocyte-macrophage colony-stimulating factors (GM-CSF or G-CSF) will accelerate regeneration. This now provides the rationale for more intensive chemotherapy schedules [3]. The injection of these growth factors has been shown to rescue several animal species from the lethal consequences of total body irradiation (TBI). For example, in dogs the use of growth factors increases survival to 50% after a lethal TBI dose of 3.5 Gy [4]. These same authors suggested that a dose-modification factor (DMF) of nearly 2 might be achieved by post-radiation intervention with growth factors. Some benefit has been reported when GM-CSF has been used in the management of radiation accident victims [5].

Rapidly renewing epithelial tissues are also controlled by growth factors, but no evidence for their potential value to modulated acute normal tissue reactions has yet emerged. There is also the potential for growth factors to ameliorate injury in late responding tissues. Some indications of growth control, in glial cell lineages, have been identified in the central nervous system (CNS) [6]. However, the development of late tissue responses involves complex cell/cell interactions and it is unlikely that the administration of one single growth factor, in isolation, would be effective. This complexity has been recognized in the various attempts that have been made to ameliorate late radiation-induced injury. A general consensus has emerged that the loss of a target cell or target cells can lead to a cascade of events prior to the expression of overt tissue damage (fig. 1). Once the cascade has been initiated, repopulation may have little relevance. The rationale for this approach is outlined in more detail elsewhere [7].

This idea is not new; it formed the basis for some earlier studies in the lung of rats by Ward et al. [8]. Such studies were initially considered to be highly unconventional because of the then dominant influence of the concept of clonogenic cell survival on the interpretation of normal tissue reactions.

```
┌─────────────────────────────────────────────────────────┐
│                                                           │
│     DIRECT AND INDIRECT EFFECT                            │
│                                                           │
│                                                           │
│        Loss of target cell(s)  ⟹  Repopulation           │
│                                                           │
│                        ⇓                                  │
│                                                           │
│     cascade reaction (reactive changes)                   │
│                                                           │
│                        ⇓                                  │
│                                                           │
│                  overt damage                             │
│              (modified tissue function)                   │
│                                                           │
└─────────────────────────────────────────────────────────┘
```

Fig. 1. Flow chart showing hypothetical direct and indirect consequence of radiation exposure leading to the late appearance of overt damage (modified tissue function). Conventional radiation-induced cell loss may lead to the development of overt damage if the cascade or reactive changes are initiated irrespective of attempts at repopulation.

The studies by Ward et al. [8, 9] showed that the loss of endothelial cells from the lung produced both time- and dose-related increases in prostacyclin (PGI_2) and thromboxane A_2 (TXA_2) expression. The greater rise in TXA_2 led to a pro-thrombotic imbalance in these two key eicosanoids. This resulted in reduced arteriole perfusion and eventually pulmonary fibrosis. The administration of penicillamine, 10 mg/day in the drinking water, reduced both PGI_2 and TXA_2 production, improved lung perfusion and reduced fibrosis [9]. The reduction in endothelial cell number, as indicated by reduced angiotensin-converting enzyme activity, was not modified.

Skin samples taken from the chest wall of animals in the same series as used for the lung studies [Ward, pers. commun.] showed that a single dose of 25 Gy produced a reduction in relative dermal thickness after 3 and 6 months (fig. 2). This effect was reduced by the daily administration of penicillamine after irradiation. Thus the action of this agent was not just restricted to reducing the eventual severity of fibrosis in an organ such as the lung, but had a wider application to other late radiation effects, mediated via an initial vascular event. Vascular changes have also been shown to be associated with a relative reduction in dermal thickness in irradiated pig skin [10].

Possible vascular mediated changes leading to a cascade of events, prior to the appearance of overt tissue damage, have provided numerous authors with a rationale for the use of different agents as prophylactic treatments in order to reduce late radiation-induced injury. Although these agents have frequently proved effective, the original rationale may have been erroneous or

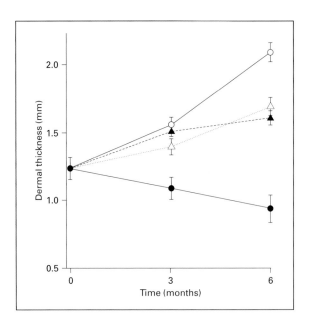

Fig. 2. Time-related changes in dermal thickness after the local irradiation of the left side of the chest wall of rats with a single dose of x-rays. The skin on the contralateral side was used as a control. Animals receiving penicillamine (10 mg/day) were compared with age-matched controls. Oral dosing was daily from the day after irradiation (penicillamine: irradiated ▲, unirradiated △; age-matched controls: irradiated ●, unirradiated ○). Error bars indicate $\pm$ SE; n = 6–10 samples [Ward, pers. commun.].

remains unproven. Pentoxifylline, a potent haemorheological agent, has been used to treat peripheral and cerebral vascular disease [11]. It has various modes of action including the ability to increase the deformability and reduce the stickiness of leucocytes, it reduces red cell aggregation and platelet adhesion, plus enhancing the release of PGI_2. Increased deformability of red cells was the rationale proposed for its use [12]. It was thought that these changes would allow freer movement of red cells through vessels narrowed by radiation. While increased red cell deformity is no longer a proven property of this agent, it was nevertheless found to reduce late dermal but not early epithelial damage to mouse skin. The DMF was approximately 1.4 when pentoxifylline was administered daily over a 30-week observation period from the first day of fractionated irradiation.

One simplistic view, for the CNS, was that a late occurring breakdown of the blood-brain barrier (BBB) resulted in oedema, reduced blood flow and fluctuating ischaemia with the possibility of problems relating to the resulting chronic reperfusion injury [13]. The use of an iron chelating agent, desferriox-

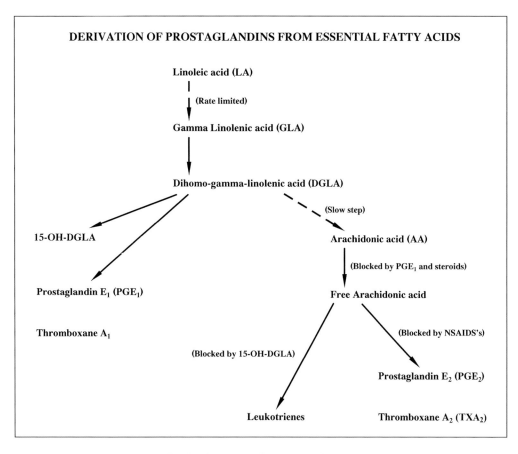

DERIVATION OF PROSTAGLANDINS FROM ESSENTIAL FATTY ACIDS

Linoleic acid (LA)

(Rate limited)

Gamma Linolenic acid (GLA)

Dihomo-gamma-linolenic acid (DGLA)

(Slow step)

15-OH-DGLA

Arachidonic acid (AA)

(Blocked by PGE$_1$ and steroids)

Prostaglandin E$_1$ (PGE$_1$)

Free Arachidonic acid

Thromboxane A$_1$

(Blocked by NSAIDS's)

(Blocked by 15-OH-DGLA)

Prostaglandin E$_2$ (PGE$_2$)

Leukotrienes

Thromboxane A$_2$ (TXA$_2$)

Fig. 3. Proposed pathways for the derivation of prostaglandins of the E$_1$ and E$_2$ series from essential fatty acids. For further explanation, see text.

amine, and a low iron diet, were seen as a means of reducing any reperfusion effects. These were not administered until 17 weeks after irradiation, when BBB breakdown was first recorded. The time of onset of radiation myelopathy was delayed and its dose-related incidence reduced. The DMF was approximately 1.1.

The concept that the loss of endothelial cells results in modified function, specifically an imbalance in the two eicosanoids PGE$_2$/PGI$_2$ and TXA$_2$, led Hopewell et al. [14, 15] to use oils containing the essential fatty acid γ-linolenic acid (GLA) as a prophylactic treatment for late radiation-induced necrosis in pig skin. GLA preferentially increases exogenous levels of prostaglandin E$_1$ (PGE$_1$). This has many desirable actions, including the down-regulation of the arachidonic acid pathway (fig. 3). It is also antiaggregatory and a potent

Table 1. Variation in ED_{50} values ($\pm$SE) for dusky/mauve erythema (DE) and dermal necrosis (N) following irradiation with single doses of $^{90}Sr/^{90}Y$ β-rays

Treatment period	Reaction type	ED_{50} ($\pm$SE)		DMF ($\pm$SE)
		So-1100	So-1129	
−4 weeks	DE	26.5±1.3	27.5±1.1	NS
−4/+16 weeks	DE	37.5±1.9	24.8±1.5	1.35±0.11
−4 weeks	N	34.8±1.4	35.0±1.5	NS
−4/+16 weeks	N	40.6±1.3	35.7±1.6	1.14±0.06

DMFs ($\pm$SE) are quoted for the difference between ED_{50} values; oils administered daily (3 ml).

vasodilator. TXA_1 produces none of the harmful side effects associated with potentially raised levels of TXA_2. An additional factor is the blocking of the production of the pro-inflammatory leukotrienes. GLA was administered to pigs daily as an oil (So-1100), 9% GLA by volume, and radiation responses were compared with those in pigs receiving a 'placebo' oil (So-1129) containing no GLA. Both oils largely consisted of linoleic acid (70–80%), the fatty acid that is a small constituent of a normal diet (fig. 3). Conversion of linoleic acid to GLA is normally rate-limited.

Oils were given either for just 4 weeks prior to irradiation or for 4 weeks prior to and 16 weeks after irradiation. The extended time period is that normally associated with the development of dermal necrosis in pig skin [15]. The presence of ischaemia (dusky/mauve erythema – DE) and/or dermal necrosis (N) can be assessed visually in pig skin and dose-effect relationships for their incidence obtained. The results obtained after the oral administration of 3 ml of oils daily are given in table 1.

Oils administered prior to irradiation had no effect; the ED_{50} values for DE and N in both groups were similar to 'non-oil' treated historical controls [15]. Continued administration of oils for 16 weeks after irradiation, over the period of the response, reduced its severity, increasing the dose needed to produce a 50% incidence of each response. DMFs of 1.35±0.11 and 1.14±0.06 were obtained for DE and N reactions, respectively.

An increase in the dose of oil administered daily after irradiation to 6 ml, i.e. both So-1100 or the 'placebo' (So-1129), general increased ED_{50} values relative to 'no-oil' controls and to daily doses of 3 ml of So-1129 (table 2). This is assumed to be due to a breakdown in the rate-limiting step when high doses of linoleic acid are administered. DMFs were significantly in excess of 1.4.

Table 2. DMFs ($\pm$SE) for the reactions of dusky/mauve erythema (DE) and dermal necrosis (N) in pig skin

Reaction	Oil type	ED$_{50}$ values $\pm$SE			DMF ($\pm$SE)
		oil (6 ml daily)		no oil	
DE	So-1100	37.97$\pm$1.82	38.21$\pm$2.76	25.56$\pm$5.66	1.49$\pm$0.35
	So-1129	38.44$\pm$2.08			
N	S0-1100	49.56$\pm$3.01	50.75$\pm$4.9	35.34$\pm$4.02	1.44$\pm$0.21
	So-1129	51.93$\pm$3.87			

Comparisons are made between the combined data for 'active' and 'placebo' (6 ml daily) and 'no oil' controls.

The assessment of late radiation-induced changes in pig skin also gave an opportunity to examine the acute reactions of erythema and moist desquamation, 3–6 weeks after irradiation. Somewhat surprisingly, an effect of the post-irradiation but not the prior irradiation administration of oil was seen. Following daily doses of 3 ml of both oils, after single doses of irradiation, a DMF of 1.24$\pm$0.06 was found, for a reduction in erythema, larger than that for moist desquamation, 1.13$\pm$0.05. 'Placebo'-related effects were again very evident when the daily oil dose was increased to 6.0 ml. The oils had a marked effect on cell proliferation in the basal layer of the pig epidermis [16].

Prophylaxis by essential fatty acid has not been limited to effects on skin. Preliminary studies in pig spinal cord have shown a reduced incidence of myelopathy after single doses of 22 Gy of ^{60}Co γ-rays [17]. In young rats, following high radiation doses, the latency for the onset of myelopathy was prolonged [18].

These experimental findings, especially those for pig skin, have resulted in the establishment of a randomized clinical study to assess the effects of fatty acids on both early and late radiation responses in human skin after post-operative radiotherapy for carcinoma of the breast. Centres in Oxford, Leeds and Cape Town were involved. The effects of an active oil (So-05057), containing both GLA and eicosapentaenoic acid (EPA), both of which suppress the E$_2$ eicosanoid pathway, were compared with a 'placebo' (So-1129). Oil, in the form of capsules (6 ml/daily), was administered for -2 to -4 weeks prior to the start of radiotherapy and for 12 weeks after the first dose fraction. Each centre was able to use its own standard radiotherapy dose

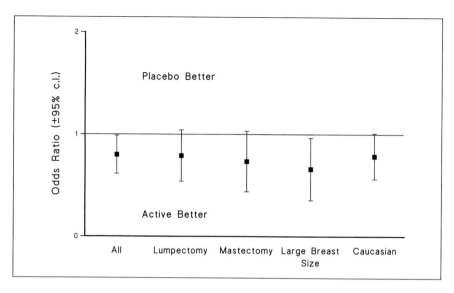

Fig. 4. Shows the odds ratio (±95% confidence interval) based on the weekly assessment of the severity of erythema in the scar site on the breast or chest wall from the state of treatment for a period of 12 weeks. The results for all patients and those of four main subgroups are shown. The ratio is always in favour of the active oil So-05057 [Scotia Pharmaceuticals Ltd, data files, pers. commun.].

fractionation schedule, a boost was almost always given to the surgical scar. Acute skin reactions were assessed over 12 weeks by visual observations.

Using megavoltage radiation, acute reactions were not severe, imposing a limitation on the study. However, in the scar site and/or in large-breasted patients, where skin doses were highest, an analysis based on the odds ratio (±95% confidence) suggested an advantage for the active group (fig. 4) for all patients (0.8 (0.64–0.99) p=0.044) and 0.67 (0.46–0.98) for patients in the subgroup, with large breasts (p=0.038).

Late changes were also assessed in these patients 78 weeks after the start of radiotherapy, or at 66 weeks after daily oral dosing with oils was withdrawn. Both the incidence and latency for the development of telangiectasia showed a significant advantage for the 'active' group (table 3).

At 78 weeks, the proportion of local recurrences, distant metastases and deaths were similar in both arms of the study (p>0.7).

Treatment

Patients who develop late radiation-induced sequelae suffer considerable discomfort. This is particularly true in cases of persistent late radiation

Table 3. Incidence and latency of telangiectasia in patients at 78 weeks after the start of radiotherapy for the treatment of carcinoma of the breast

Telangiectasia	Treatment group		p value
	active	placebo	
Incidence, %	34.5	47.2	0.04
Latency, weeks	80.1	77.9	0.04

Source: Scotia Pharmaceuticals Ltd database (with permission).
Patients received an active oil (So-05057) or placebo oil (So-1129) for 12 weeks after the start of radiotherapy.

necrosis in soft tissue. Pilot studies with pentoxifylline [19] showed a high healing rate (87%) in 15 patients selected for the study on the basis that conventional methods of treatment had failed. A subgroup of 8 of the cases also had significant pain. This was ameliorated within 3–8 weeks of starting treatment. The theory was that healing of the necrosis was initiated by an improvement in the microcirculation around the wound; the rate of healing was also clearly related to the initial size of the lesion. This was not a placebo-controlled study; indeed such studies may present ethical issues as will be discussed later.

Fibrosis and/or tissue scarring can also be deleterious to patients as a late consequence of radiotherapy. In a series of experimental studies in pigs [20], the effects of very high doses of radiation, as encountered in accidents involving the skin and subcutaneous tissues, were examined. Although of interest, these studies do not directly relate to radiotherapeutic problems, unless tissue breakdown and subsequent scarring was a feature of a specific radiotherapy case. The efficacy of liposomal superoxide dismutase (Cu/Zn-SOD or Mn-SOD) on the regression of a block of fibrotic tissue in the thigh muscle of pigs was assessed relative to a control group. The block of fibrotic tissue was induced as a consequence of irradiation with a large single dose of 160 Gy of ^{192}Ir γ-rays. This high dose produced an extensive volume of subcutaneous and cutaneous necrosis within 3 weeks, healing was slow, but was complete within 26 weeks. This left a surface scar and a substantial block of fibrous tissue in the muscle. A limited number of subcutaneous injections of liposomal SOD produced significant regression of the block of fibrotic tissue over 12 weeks. This phenomenon is not fully understood.

Clinical studies have also been undertaken with Cu/Zn-SOD [21]. Thirty-four patients with 42 distinct, palpable, zones of long-standing radiation-induced fibrosis were treated over 3 weeks with twice-weekly intramuscular injections of 5 mg of Liposod. In most patients, regression of the fibrosis had begun during the third week of treatment and was maximum after 8 weeks. It was suggested that SOD, as an antioxidant, may act as an anti-inflammatory drug. However, it seemed to be equally effective in what was termed inflammatory fibrosis as compared with 'cold' fibrosis. Additional, more controlled, studies are needed to evaluate the full potential of SOD.

Towards Clinical Trials with Pharmacological Agents

Although the mechanisms underlying the modulation of radiation-induced damage in experiment studies are uncertain, the potential for such approaches are now obvious. Indeed, a limited number of clinical studies have already been undertaken and positive results obtained. The design of future trials poses some problems and requires some complex choices.

Prophylaxis versus Treatment Trials
There are two fundamentally different approaches to testing a modulator of radiation-induced normal tissue damage. In an attempt to prevent the injury from occurring, drugs can be used from the time of irradiation (a prophylactic approach), or it can be used to treat injury after it develops (a treatment approach). The trial with EFAs is an example of a prophylactic approach, whereas the pentoxifylline study represented a treatment approach. There are advantages and disadvantages to each approach.
Prophylactic trials take advantage of the fact that the agents tested so far are most effective when given early in the development of the injury. This has the disadvantage that many patients must be treated in order to prevent injuries in an unidentified subpopulation. If these trials are based on the prevention of severe normal tissue injuries, they will require a very large number of patients and a long follow-up, and hence may be expensive. An alternative approach would be to use a graded assessment of normal tissue toxicity; while the lower grades of injury might be of only minor clinical significance, such an approach would both require fewer patients and have the potential for benefiting a larger number of them.
Treatment trials have the advantage that only patients who have developed the injury need to be treated, thereby reducing the size and cost of the trial. There may also be an ethical problem with some randomized treatment trials. On the other hand, nonrandomized treatment trials may not be viewed as experimental if they are done with agents known from experimental studies to have some treatment efficacy for the injury.

Toxicity Reduction vs. Radiation Dose Escalation

When a modulator of radiation-induced damage is tested there are two fundamentally different trial designs. The modifier can be used with standard radiotherapy, in an attempt to reduce normal tissue toxicity, or it can be used with higher doses, in an attempt to improve the therapeutic ratio (dose escalation).

The conservative approach would be to use potential modifiers to decrease the incidence or severity of normal tissue complications. However, this approach is limited by the fact that complication rates for many types of radiotherapy are so low that improvements would be difficult to prove. The advantage of this approach is that if the modulator fails to work, relatively little is lost, provided that the modulator itself produces only minimal toxicity.

A more aggressive approach would be to combine the use of modifiers with more intensive radiotherapy. This is a theoretically attractive approach, as the steepness of the tumour control dose-response relationship is such that a 10–20% increase in dose would be expected to lead to a detectable increase in tumour control rates in many sites [22]. However, as an initial approach this would be risky, since the failure of the modifier could lead to a dramatic rise in complication rates.

Thus a practical compromise is to initially use modulators to decrease complication rates, and to simultaneously establish the safety of the approach. Even if a statistically significant decrease in complication rates could not be demonstrated in such trials, they would pave the way for gradual radiation dose escalation. This represents a new challenge for radiotherapy into the next century.

Acknowledgements

The author thanks Dr. William F. Ward for permission to use previously unpublished data and to Ms. Kate Scott, Scotia Pharmaceuticals Ltd, for the use of results from their database. Mrs. Margaret Staff is also thanked for the typing of the manuscript.

References

1   Overgaard J, Sand Hansen H, Andersen AP, Hjelm-Hansen M, Jorgensen K, Sandberg E, Berthelsen A, Hammer R, Pedersen M: Misonidazole combined with split-course radiotherapy in the treatment of invasive carcinoma of larynx and pharynx: Report from the DAHANCA 2 study. Int J Radiat Oncol Biol Phys 1989;16:1065–1068.
2   Blumberg AL, Nelson DF, Gramkowski M, Glover DJ, Glick JH, Yuhaas J, Kligerman MM: Clinical trials of WR2721 with radiation therapy. Int J Radiat Oncol Biol Phys 1982;8:561–563.
3   Bronchud MH, Scarffe JH, Thatcher N, Crowther D, Souza LM, Alton NK, Testa NG, Dexter TM: Phase 1/11 study of recombinant human granulocyte colony-stimulating intensive chemotherapy for small cell lung cancer. Br J Cancer 1987;56:809–813.

4   Baverstock KF, Papworth DG, Townsend KMS: Man's sensitivity to bone marrow failure follows whole-body exposure to low LET irradiation: Inferences to be drawn from animal experiments. Int J Radiat Biol 1985;45:397–411.

5   Butturini AB, de Souza PC, Gale RP, Cordiero JM, Lopes DM, Neto C, Cunha CB, de Souza CEP, Ho WG, Tabak DG, Sanpai JM, Burla A: Use of recombinant GM-CSF in the Brazil radiation accident. Lancet 1988;ii:471.

6   Hanley MR: Peptide regulatory factors in the nervous system. Lancet 1989;i:1373–1376.

7   Hopewell JW: Rational and clinical advantage to be obtained from the therapeutic modulation of normal tissue injury; in Hagen V, Harder D, Jung H, Streffer C (eds): Radiation Research 1895–1995. Würzburg, Sturtz, 1985, vol 2, pp 882–885.

8   Ward WF, Molteni A, Solliday NH, Jones GE: The relationship between endothelial cell dysfunction and collagen accumulation in irradiated rat lung. Int J Radiat Oncol Biol Phys 1985;11:1985–1990.

9   Ward WF, Molteni A, Ts'a C, Solliday NH: Functional response of the pulmonary endothelium to thoracic irradiation in rats: Differential modification by D-penicillamine. Int J Radiat Oncol Biol Phys 1987;13:1505–1513.

10 Rezvani M, Hamlet R, Hopewell JW, Sieber VK: Time and dose-related changes in the thickness of pig skin after irradiation with single doses of ^{90}Sr/^{90}Y β-rays. Int J Radiat Biol 1994;65:497–502.

11 Hopewell JW, Calvo W, Jaenke R, Reinhold HS, Robbins MEC, Whitehouse E: Microcirculation and radiation damage; in Hinkelbein W, Bruggmoser G, Frommhold H, Wannermacher M (eds): Acute and Long-Term Side-Effects of Radiotherapy. Recent Res Cancer Res 1993;130:1–16.

12 Dion MW, Hussey DH, Osborne JW: The effect of pentoxifylline on early and late radiation injury following fractionated irradiation in C3H mice. Int J Radiat Oncol Biol Phys 1989;17:101–107.

13 Hornsey S, Myers R, Jenkinson T: The reduction of radiation damage to the spinal cord by post-irradiation administration of vasoactive drugs. Int J Radiat Oncol Biol Phys 1990;18:1437–1442.

14 Hopewell JW, Robbins MEC, van den Aardweg GJMJ, Morris GM, Ross GA, Whitehouse E, Horrobin DF, Scott CA: The modulation of radiation-induced damage to pig skin by essential fatty acids. Br J Cancer 1993;68:1–7.

15 Hopewell JW, van den Aardweg GJMJ, Morris GM, Rezvani M, Robbins MEC, Ross GA, Whitehouse EM, Scott CA, Horrobin DF: Amelioration of both early and late radiation-induced damage to pig skin by essential fatty acids. Int J Radiat Oncol Biol Phys 1994;30:1119–1125.

16 Morris GM, Hopewell JW, Ross GA, Whitehouse E, Wilding D, Scott CA: Trophic effects of essential fatty acids on pig skin. Cell Prolif 1995;28:73–84.

17 Hopewell JW, van den Aardweg GJMJ, Morris GM, Rezvani M, Robbins MEC, Ross GA, Whitehouse EM: Unsaturated lipids as modulators of radiation damage in normal tissues; in Horrobin DF (ed): New Approaches to Cancer Therapy: Unsaturated Lipids and Photodynamic Therapy. London, Churchill Communications, 1994, pp 88–108.

18 El-Agamawi AY, Hopewell JW, Plowman PN, Rezvani M, Wilding D: Modulation of normal tissue response to radiation. Br J Radiol 1996;69:374–375.

19 Dion MW, Hussey DH, Doornbos JF, Vigliotti AP, Wen BC, Anderson B: Preliminary results of a pilot study of pentoxifylline in the treatment of late radiation soft tissue necrosis. Int J Radiat Oncol Biol Phys 1990;19:401–407.

20 Lefaix JL, Delanian S, Leplat JJ, Tricaud Y, Martin M, Nimrod A, Baillet F, Daburon F: Successful treatment of radiation-induced fibrosis using Cu/Zn-SOD and Mn-Sod: An experimental study. Int J Radiat Oncol Biol Phys 1996;35:302–312.

21 Delanian S, Baillet F, Huart J, Lefaix JL, Maulard C, Housset M: Successful treatment of radiation-induced fibrosis using liposomal Cu/Zn superoxide dismutase: Clinical trial. Radiother Oncol 1994;32:12–20.

22 Thames HD, Schultheiss TE, Hendry JH, Tucker SL, Dubray BM, Brock WA: Can modest escalations of dose be detected as increased tumor control. Int J Radiat Oncol Biol Phys 1992;22:241–246.

John Hopewell, Normal Tissue Radiobiology Group, Research Institute,
University of Oxford, Churchill Hospital, Oxford OX3-7LJ (UK)

Meyer JL (ed): Radiation Injury. Advances in Management and Prevention.
Front Radiat Ther Oncol. Basel, Karger, 1999, vol 32, pp 21–33

··························

Radiation-Induced Eye Injury from Head and Neck Therapy

Rodney R. Million, James T. Parsons

Department of Radiation Oncology, University of Florida College of Medicine,
Gainesville, Fla., USA

> *The most feared illness is blindness;*
> *the second most feared is cancer.*
>
> Reader's Digest Poll

The various structures of the eye and periorbital tissues, including the optic nerve, have different tolerance levels to radiation. When these tissues must be irradiated in their entirety or in part, the patient is at risk for developing sequelae, some of which can be devastating. While this paper will discuss the radiation response of each of the tissues separately, all or some of the processes may be occurring at the same time, depending on tissues included in the irradiated area. The tissues at risk differ widely, depending on whether one is treating a simple skin cancer of the eyelid compared to an advanced paranasal sinus cancer with extension of tumor into the orbit.

The objective of the radiation oncologist is to minimize eye injury through knowledge of the normal tissue limits for each structure. Even if it is likely that blindness will occur in one eye, an attempt should be made to preserve the eyeball for cosmetic reasons as a prosthesis seldom stays in place after high-dose radiotherapy. It is essential to consult a knowledgeable ophthalmologist before irradiation to assist in the management of problems that occur during the course of treatment as well as during follow-up. The ophthalmologist may be able to predict an increased risk for some types of injury so that the radiation oncologist may be able to reduce the dose or add additional ocular protection to prevent certain problems. Concurrent diseases (such as diabetes) or drug therapy (both chemotherapeutic and nonchemotherapeutic) may enhance the radiation effect on the eye and optic nerve.

Table 1. Radiation therapy (RT) cataract (43 adults, 85 eyes) [from 16]

Status	Eyes, n	Dose range[1], Gy
No RT cataract	69	0.45–12.60
Possible RT cataract	12	1.00–13.75
Stationary cataract	2	20.40–27.10
Progressive cataract	2	35.70–39.00

[1] Treatments reconstructed on adult cadavers; predominantly supervoltage.

Eyelids and Lacrimal Ducts

The eyelids and lacrimal ducts are normally at risk only in patients with skin cancers in and about the eyelids in which high doses are confined to the lid with shielding of the remainder of the eyeball. Loss of lashes is to be expected. With treatment of larger and more advanced cancers involving the lid margin, ectropion or entropion may develop and may require surgical correction. The lacrimal apparatus, whether involved by tumor or incidentally irradiated, may becomme obstructed. (See chapter by Gordon on management of the sequelae of eye complications.)

Cataracts

Relatively low doses may result in radiation cataracts, but the exact doses and the time to occurrence are not finely tuned. Merriam et al. [13] stated that with doses of 2.0–6.5 Gy of fractionated external beam radiation, a third of the patients experienced progressive opacities, whereas following a dose of 6.5–11.5 Gy, only one third had stationary opacities. The latent time to development of opacities was shortened by increasing doses. For a group receiving 2.5–6.5 Gy, the average time in which cataracts were first discovered was 8 years 7 months. In the group exposed to 6.51–11.5 Gy, the time to discovery of the cataract was 4 years 4 months.

Contrary to the above information, a series reported by Parker et al. [16] showed a different dose response to fractionated radiotherapy in patients treated for paranasal sinus tumors (table 1).

Depending on the radiation dose and fractionation, a cataract may remain stationary at any stage and produce little or no visual impairment. On the other hand, it may become a mature cataract, indistinguishable from other cataracts, and result in complete blindness. Several patients from the University of Florida series did not develop cataracts until 3.0–3.5 years afters 40–70 Gy to the lens with fractionated external beam radiation.

Management of Radiation-Induced Cataracts

Radiation-induced cataracts may be treated by cataract removal. If dry-eye syndrome is not associated with the cataract, a contact lens may be used satisfactorily. Intraocular lens implant is apparently safe following low doses of radiation.

After moderate doses (e.g. as for lymphomas), one would consider an extraction of the cataract if preservation of vision is probable or there is a reason to examine the retina. For instance, a patient who has received 45 Gy in 25 fractions would be on the border of developing radiation retinopathy. Removal of the cataract would allow determination of residual vision and whether or not treatment of radiation-induced retinopathy by panretinal laser might be warranted to save the eye.

After high-dose radiotherapy (e.g. 60 Gy or higher), the risk for radiation retinopathy and optic neuropathy increases, and removal of the cataract would only be justified to attempt to treat radiation retinopathy to avoid closed-angle glaucoma.

Our limited experience with intraocular lens implantation has not been spectacular. Implants were performed at 2, 2.5 and 4 years after 51, 35 and 60 Gy to the entire eye. The major lacrimal gland had been shielded in each case. The first patient required reoperation to replace a dislocated lens and eventually required a conjunctival flap to relieve pain from the keratopathy; all useful vision was lost. Visual acuity in the second patient returned to 20/15 with no operative complications after 35 Gy. The third patient never achieved better than 20/200 visual acuity; in addition, postoperative keratopathy developed in the eye. Newer techniques for intraocular lens implantation might be safer.

Dry-Eye Syndrome

Tears are composed of secretions from the lacrimal gland and accessory lacrimal glands located in the upper and lower eyelid. The accessory lacrimal glands are found predominantly in the upper lid and are responsible for basal tear flow. Tears from the major lacrimal gland are brought into use in more extreme situations.

Figure 1 and table 2 and 3 show the risks for dry-eye syndrome according to dose when all lacrimal tissues are irradiated. The dose at which dry-eye syndrome begins to occur is about 30 Gy, and the incidence increases to 100%

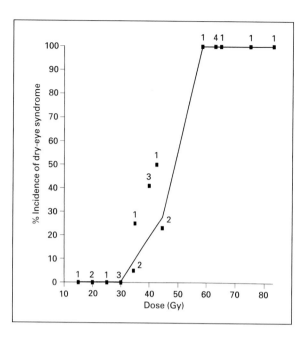

Fig. 1. Sigmoid dose-response curve for production of dry-eye complications. Points are numbered to correspond with authors: (1) Parsons et al. [19]; (2) Bessell et al. [3]; (3) Letschert et al. [11]; and (4) Morita and Kawabe [15]. Dose ranges are shown in tables 2 and 3. [Data from 19, p. 779, fig. 3.]

at 55–60 Gy. There seems to be no difference in the risk in relation to age, but the data are sparse.

The dry-eye syndrome develops within a few months after radiotherapy so that in the majority of patients, corneal vascularization is often pronounced by 9 months. Three patients did not develop it for 4–11 years after doses ≤30–45 Gy. Two of these 3 patients had also received chemotherapy. Twelve of the 20 patients who developed dry-eye syndrome required removal of the eye for control of symptoms.

In the early years when the orbit was involved, it was thought that the entire orbit was at risk for subclinical extension that could not be diagnosed by available imaging techniques. However, with today's imaging refinements, involvement of the floor or medial portion of the orbit does not preclude sparing of the lacrimal gland and at least part of the upper lid. Shielding of the lacrimal gland is merely a matter of design. Sparing of the upper lid can be increased by the use of a lid retractor, which moves the upper lid to a more superior postion so it can be shielded along with the lacrimal gland.

Table 2. Incidence of severe dry-eye syndrome according to total dose (University of Florida data)[1] [from 19, p. 778, table 3]

Dose range, Gy	Incidence	
	n	%
10–20	0/4	0
20.01–30	0/2	0
30.01–40	2/8	25
40.01–45	1/2	50
45.01–56.99	No data	
57–60	3/3	100
60.01–70	5/5	100
70.01–80	8/8	100
80.01–83	1/1	100

[1] Data shown in figure 1.

Table 3. Incidence of severe dry-eye syndrome according to total dose [from 19, p. 779, table 5]

Author[1]	Dose, Gy	Incidence	
		n	%
(2) Bessell et al. [3]	< 30	0/17	0
	30–39	2/43	5
	40–49	3/13	23
(3) Letschert et al. [11]	30	0/3	0
	40	9/22	41
(4) Morita and Kawabe [15]	63	3/3	100

[1] Numbers preceding authors' names correspond to numbered points in figure 1.

Radiation Retinopathy

Radiation retinopathy presents a clinical picture similar to that seen in diabetic retinopathy. Patients with diabetes and small vessel occlusive disease are at increased risk of radiation reinopathy. There is usually a delay of 1.5–3.0 years from the time of irradiation to the expression of the syndrome, during which visual acuity usually remains normal. The retinopathy may be confined

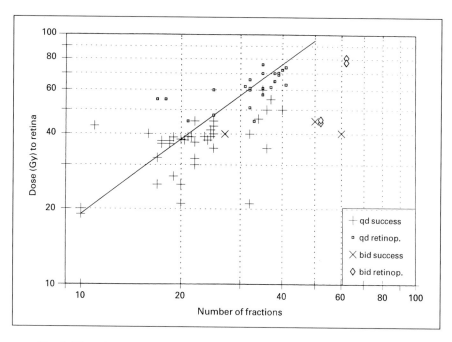

Fig. 2. Time-dose scatter distribution of radiation retinopathy after external beam irradiation. The reference line represents treatment at 1.9 Gy/fraction. qd = Once a day; bid = twice a day. [Data from 17, p. 769, fig. 3.]

to the retina with deterioration of vision. About half the patients proceed to rubeosis iridis with the secondary effect of closed-angle glaucoma.

Figure 2 and table 4 show the dose response for the production of radiation retinopathy for 64 patients. In the patients who developed retinopathy in the 45–49 Gy region, 1 of the patients also had received chemotherapy, and 2 of the patients had diabetes. Only 7 patients included in table 4 had been irradiated with twice-a-day fractionation; 2 of 3 patients in whom the retina received 46 Gy in approximately 52 fractions developed retinopathy (1 was diabetic). The data for twice-a-day fractionation are too limited to reach a conclusion.

There was no relationship between age and the risk for retinopathy. Seven patients received chemotherapy in conjunction with radiation therapy (table 5).

A number of reports have implicated diabetes as a factor increasing the risk for retinopathy [1, 4, 7, 20]. Several publications have implicated concurrent chemotherapy or chemotherapy in close proximity to radiation as a risk factor for retinopathy [4, 5, 12, 14]. Data from the Intergroup Rhabdomyosarcoma Study (IRS I) in relation to radiotherapy plus chemotherapy are confusing [10]. A review of the discussion by Parsons et al. [17] is recommended.

Table 4. Incidence of vision loss due to radiation retinopathy according to dose and dose per fraction (68 eyes in 64 patients) [from 17, p. 770, table 4]

Dose, Gy	Dose (Gy) per fraction		
	<1.9	≥1.9	Total
<30	0/5	0/2	0.7
30–39.99	0/10	0/6	0/16
40–44.99	0/8	0/2	0/10
45–49.99	3/6	2/3	5/9
50–54.99	1/3	No data	1/3
55–59.99	1/2	2/2	3/4
60–64.99	4/5	3/3	7/8
65–69.99	2/2	1/1	3/3
70–74.99	4/4	1/1	5/5
>75	2/2	1/1	3/3

Table 5. Retinopathy: radiotherapy plus chemotherapy (University of Florida series) [from 17]

Dose, Gy	Fractions, n	Patients, n
Without retinopathy		
32	17	1
40	16–25	4
With retinopathy		
45[1]	21	1
51	32	1

[1] The risk was 4 of 10 at 45–51 Gy without chemotherapy.

Management of Radiation-Induced Retinopathy

Some success has been reported with panretinal laser therapy of neovascular tissues. Patients should have close follow-up so that this therapy may be applied before major visual loss occurs.

The Optic Nerve

Optic neuropathy is divided into anterior optic neuropathy and retrobulbar optic neuropathy, but for practical purposes the syndromes are essentially

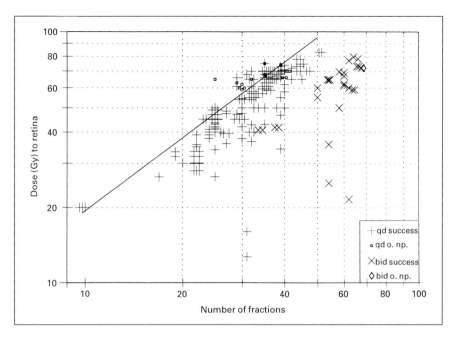

Fig. 3. Optic nerve dose vs. number of fractions for optic nerve injury secondary to irradiation. The reference line represents treatment at 1.9 Gy/fraction. qd = Once a day; bid = twice a day; o.np. = optic neuropathy. [Data from 18, p. 759, fig. 3.]

the same except that the physical findings in retrobulbar optic neuropathy may take longer to appear following the loss of vision. Although onset is usually from 1 to 5 years, 3 cases have been observed to occur after more than 5 years, and 1 occurred as long as 14 years after irradiation. Patients usually present with a field defect that progresses to blindness. Some patients may appear with sudden blindness.

Figure 3 and tables 6 and 7 demonstrate the dose response. Optic neuropathy is sensitive to dose per fraction (table 6) and was noted in our series only in patients over the age of 50 (table 7). Patients 50 years of age or younger had a high tolerance to damage of the optic nerve even with doses in excess of 65 Gy. Patients with preexisting small vessel occlusive disease are probably at increased risk.

Magnetic resonance imaging (MRI) has recently been demonstrated to aid in the diagnosis and to help rule out neoplasm as a cause. T1-weighted MR with gadolinium and T2-weighted images will show an enhancing nerve consistent with optic neuropathy. The nerve will be slightly enlarged. If the MRI is repeated some months later, this enhancement may disappear.

Table 6. Optic neuropathy according to optic nerve dose, fractionation scheme, and dose per fractionation [from 18, p. 760, table 4]

Dose range, Gy	Dose per fraction, Gy		
	once a day		twice a day[c]
	<1.9 Gy[a]	≥1.9 Gy[b]	
<30	0/7	0/3	0/2
30–39.99	0/25	No data	0/1
40–49.99	0/34	0/4	0/4
50–54.99	0/10	0/1	0/1
55–59.99	0/15	1/1	0/3
60–64.99	0/6	4/6	0/7
65–69.99	2/24	4/10	0/3
70–74.99	3/27	1/7	1/4
≥75	0/4	0/1	0/4

Median and mean lengths of follow-up: [a] 8 and 7.5 years; [b] 13 and 11 years; [c] 4 and 4 years.

Table 7. Optic neuropathy according to age and total dose [from 18, p. 760, table 5]

Dose range, Gy	Age at time of treatment, years			
	<20	20–50	51–70[1]	>70[2]
55–55.99	0/1	0/9	1/6 (17%)	0/3
60–64.99	0/1	0/5	1/9 (11%)	3/4 (75%)
65–69.99	No data	0/14	3/15 (20%)	3/8 (38%)
70–74.99	No data	0/7	2/27 (7%)	3/4 (75%)
≥75	0/2	0/3	1/5 (20%)	No data
Total	0/4	0/38	8/62 (13%)	9/19 (47%)

[1] Optic nerve doses in Gy (fraction size in Gy) in injured patients (51–70 years old): 59 (1.97); 62 (2.07); 67 (1.91); 68 (1.94); 65 (2.03); 72 (1.06); 70 (1.75); 75 (2.14).

[2] Optic nerve doses in Gy (fraction size in Gy) in injured patients (>70 years old): 60 (2); 60 (2); 63 (2.17); 66 (1.65); 66 (1.65); 65 (2.6); 70 (1.71); 70 (1.71); 74.25 (1.9).

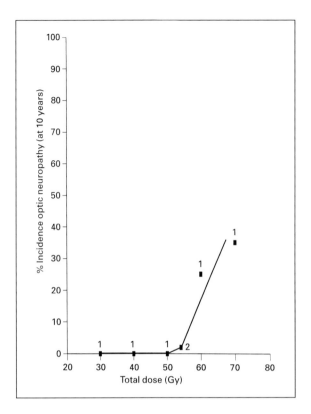

Fig. 4. Dose-response data from the (1) University of Florida [18] and the (2) University of California at San Francisco [9] for the development of optic neuropathy. [Data from 18, p. 762, fig. 5.]

Chemotherapy may sensitize the optic nerve to injury. There are reports of optic neuropathy occurring after doses in a range of 40–49 Gy at 2 Gy/fraction, or lower radiation doses when chemotherapy was given concurrently or sequentially [2, 6, 8, 21]. Vincristine, vincristine plus multiple other drugs, and oral CCNU have been implicated as increased risk factors for optic neuropathy in conjunction with radiotherapy [18].

Figure 4 shows a dose-response curve at 10 years for patients who received ≤2 Gy/fraction. The data from Goldsmith et al. [9] showed 1 patient developing optic neuropathy after 54 Gy at 1.8 Gy/fraction.

Management of Optic Nerve Injury

No proven therapy exists for this problem. Hyperbaric therapy and steroids have been tried without success. Prevention of this problem is aimed at controlling the dose level to the optic nerve by careful treatment planning. In particular, one should avoid the use of anterior electron fields that aim between the eyeballs to increase the dose to disease in this area. Electrons delivered in this manner produce areas of high dose centered in the optic nerves because of the scatter pattern that occurs with the irregular contour created by the nose.

Guidelines for Prevention of Radiation-Induced Eye Injury

The following guidelines are suggested in order to reduce the risk of eye complications:

(1) Involve the ophthalmologist early; arrange continued follow-up of the patient during treatment and afterwards to help manage and perhaps prevent sequelae.
(2) Double shield the contralateral eye to reduce transit radiation.
(3) Spare lacrimal tissue with use of: (a) a lacrimal gland shield; (b) a lid retractor to spare lid treatment; (c) field reductions.
(4) Aggressively manage all anterior segment complications to avoid perforation and infection.
(5) Consider surgical resection (e.g. craniofacial resections) to reduce the tumor burden so that the dose used for postoperative irradiation may fall within the safety margin.
(6) Recognize the tolerance dose of the various tissues. Doses ≤ 1.9 Gy/fraction have generally reduced the risk of sequelae. Twice-a-day radiotherapy has shown promise in reducing the risk for optic neuropathy.
(7) Treat all fields in each therapy session.
(8) Instruct the patient to gaze straight ahead with the eyes open and not to turn the eyes to one side or the other.
(9) Cylindrical eye blocks have been used to shield the central portion of the eyeball and are successful in avoiding eye complications. However, the cylinder and its penumbra may shield tumor. There are no data to answer this conundrum.
(10) Reduce field sizes when possible at 40–45 Gy.
(11) Evaluate retinal function before cataract extraction when doses were above the tolerance level of the retina and optic nerve.
(12) Decisions about cataract extraction should be made in consultation with the ophthalmologist (e.g. advisability of an intraocular lens).
(13) Consider use of panretinal laser photocoagulation, which may prevent neovascular complications and maintain a cosmetically acceptable eye.
(14) Try to preserve the eye even if vision is lost. The orbit will not tolerate a prosthesis after high-dose radiotherapy.

(15) Avoid using an anterior electron field in the treatment of masses centered between the orbits.

(16) Obtain a very specific informed consent from the patient and dictate it separately into the chart. The patient should be well informed of the consequences of radiation treatment in or about the eye. It is preferable to explain these consequences in the presence of not only the patient, but also one or more family members, and to repeat the information at least once to assure yourself that everyone understands the risk. The patient may certainly want to participate in a decision about the relative risks of cancer recurrence and blindness and to be involved in selecting doses.

O loss of sight, of thee I most complain!
Blind among enemies, O worse than chains,
Dungeons, or beggary, or decrepit age!
John Milton: Samson Agonistes

A blind man leaned against a wall;
– 'This is the boundary of the world' he said.
Proverb

References

1 Amoaku WM, Archer DB: Cephalic radiation and retinal vasculopathy. Eye 1990;4:195–203.
2 Appen RE, Bosch A: Bilateral loss of vision following radiation therapy. Neuroophthalmology 1983;3:97–102.
3 Bessell EM, Henck JM, Whitelocke RA, Wright JE: Ocular morbidity after radiotherapy of orbital and conjunctival lymphoma. Eye 1987;1:90–96.
4 Brown GC, Shields JA, Sanborn G, Augsburger JJ, Savino PJ, Schatz NJ: Radiation retinopathy. Opthalmology 1982;89:1494–1501.
5 Chan RC, Shukovsky LJ: Effects of irradiation on the eye. Radiology 1976;120:673–675.
6 Choi KN, Rotman M, Aziz H, Potters L, Stark R, Rosenthal JC: Locally advanced paranasal sinus and nasopharynx tumors treated with hyperfractionated radiation and concomitant infusion cisplatin. Cancer 1991;67:2748–2752.
7 Dhir SP, Joshi AV, Banerjee AK: Radiation retinopathy in diabetes mellitus: Report of a case. Acta Radiol Oncol 1982;21:111–113.
8 Fishman ML, Bean SC, Cogan DG: Optic atrophy following prophylactic chemotherapy and cranial radiation for acute lymphocytic leukemia. Am J Ophthalmol 1976;82:571–576.
9 Goldsmith BJ, Rosenthal SA, Wara WM, Larson DA: Optic neuropathy after irradiation of meningioma. Radiology 1992;185:71–76.
10 Heyn R, Ragab A, Raney RB Jr, Ruymann F, Tefft M, Lawrence W Jr, Soule E, Maurer HM: Late effects of therapy in orbital rhabdomyosarcoma in children. A report from the Intergroup Rhabdomyosarcoma Study. Cancer 1986;57:1738–1743.
11 Letschert JGJ, Gonzalez-Gonzalez D, Oskam J, Koornneef L, van Dijk JD, Boukes R, Bras J, van Heerde P, Bartelink H: Results of radiotherapy in patients with stage I orbital non-Hodgkin's lymphoma. Radiother Oncol 1991;22:36–44.
12 Lopez PF, Sternberg P Jr, Dabbs CK, Vogler WR, Crocker I, Kalin NS: Bone marrow transplant retinopathy. Am J Ophthalmol 1991;112:635–646.

13   Merriam GR Jr, Szechter A, Focht EF: The effects of ionizing radiations on the eye. Front Radiat Ther Oncol. Basel, Karger, 1972, vol 6, pp 346–385.

14   Mewis L, Tang RS, Salmonsen PC: Radiation retinopathy after 'safe' levels of irradiation. Invest Ophthalmol Vis 1982;22:222.

15   Morita K, Kawabe Y: Late effects on the eye of conformation radiotherapy for carcinoma of the paranasal sinuses and nasal cavity. Radiology 1979;130:227–232.

16   Parker RG, Burnett LL, Wootton P et al: Radiation cataracts in clinical therapeutic radiology. Radiology 1964;82:794–799.

17   Parsons JT, Bova FJ, Fitzgerald CR, Mendenhall WM, Million RR: Radiation retinopathy after external-beam irradiation: Analysis of time-dose factors. Int J Radiat Oncol Biol Phys 1994;30: 765–773.

18   Parsons JT, Bova FJ, Fitzgerald CR, Mendenhall WM, Million RR: Radiation optic neuropathy after megavoltage external-beam irradiation: Analysis of time-dose factors. Int J Radiat Oncol Biol Phys 1994;30:755–763.

19   Parsons JT, Bova FJ, Fitzgerald CR, Mendenhall WM, Million RR: Severe dry-eye syndrome following external beam irradiation. Int J Radiat Oncol Biol Phys 1994;30:775–780.

20   Viebahn M, Barricks ME, Osterloh MD: Synergism between diabetic and radiation retinopathy: Case report and review. Br J Ophthalmol 1991;75:629–632.

21   Wilson WB, Perez GM, Kleinschmidt-Demasters BK: Sudden onset of blindness in patients treated with oral CCNU and low-dose cranial irradiation. Cancer 1987;59:901–907.

James T. Parsons, MD, Department of Radiation Oncology,
PO Box 100385, Gainesville, FL 32610-0385 (USA)

Meyer JL (ed): Radiation Injury. Advances in Management and Prevention.
Front Radiat Ther Oncol. Basel, Karger, 1999, vol 32, pp 34–48

....

Current Concepts in the Management of Oral/Dental Adverse Sequelae of Head and Neck Radiotherapy

Sol Silverman, Jr.

School of Dentistry, University of California, San Francisco, Calif., USA

Radiation Effects

Ionizing radiation delivered in doses that will kill cancer cells induces unavoidable changes in the surrounding normal tissues, causing compromises in function and host defenses and severe complications [1–4]. Intraoral changes include acute mucositis (erythema, pseudomembrane-covered ulcerations, and hyperkeratosis). Epithelial ulcerations may become so severe as to require a temporary break in treatment to allow repair. Analgetic, antibiotic and anti-inflammatory medications can be helpful for both signs and symptoms. There is also a risk for posttreatment delayed soft tissue necrosis, which may not occur for months or even years. Damage to the bone can result in osteonecrosis and sequestration or progressive osteonecrosis. Radiation changes in the salivary glands result in abnormal saliva (hyposalivation, xerostomia) and secondarily increased caries and other dental defects. Radiation also directly damages the taste buds in the tongue and results in transient, or sometimes permanent, loss or alteration of taste (dysgeusia, ageusia).

Radiation effects on chromosomes (mutagenesis) may predispose cells to subsequent malignant behavior. However, this is usually a long-term effect, which therefore has not been a significant threat or complication in treating adults with head and neck cancers. The loss of salivary protection (quantity and quality) against carcinogens may increase risks for epithelial neoplasia, particularly in those patients who continue to smoke [5].

Mucocutaneous Changes
Unless intraoral or interstitial treatment is used, most patients will develop some erythema and moderate tanning of the skin in the treatment portal.

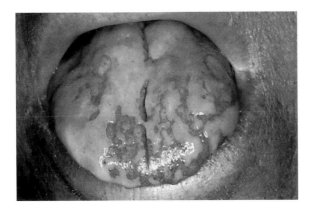

Fig. 1. Severe mucositis of tongue during the fourth week of radiotherapy (approx. 4,000 cGy).

Hair follicles are quite radiosensitive, therefore if hair is in the treatment beam it will cease to grow and will fall out. This is often transient.

The acute oral mucosal reaction (mucositis) is secondary to radiation-induced mitotic death of the basal cells in the oral mucosa. Because these cells require 2 weeks to mature, there is a delay of about this time between the onset of radiation therapy and the appearance of mucositis. If the radiation is delivered at a rate equivalent to the ability of the oral mucosa to regenerate, then only mild mucositis will be seen. When the weekly or daily dose is increased just slightly, destruction (necrosis) will outpace proliferation and a rather marked mucositis will develop (fig. 1). This occurs at daily doses >180 cGy. Acute mucositis is not related to late radiation-induced atrophy and telangiectasis of the mucosa (fig. 2). This late change often increases the risk for pain and/or necrosis. Smoking has been associated as a co-factor in worsening acute mucositis reactions.

Management of acute mucositis may sometimes require a 1-week interruption of therapy. Topical anesthetics (viscous xylocaine) may be of some value, but the pain usually requires systemic analgetic drugs, sometimes at the level of morphine [6, 7]. Since infections may be associated, appropriate diagnosis and antimicrobial agents must be considered for either fungal or bacterial organisms. Viral infections are rarely a complication of radiation-induced mucositis. A short course of systemic prednisone (40–80 mg daily for not more than 1 week) has been helpful in reducing inflammation and discomfort.

Loss of Taste

Taste buds, which occur primarily in the circumvallate and fungiform papillae, are very sensitive to radiation. Because of their location in the tongue,

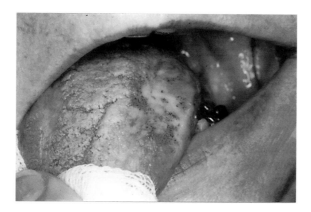

Fig. 2. Telangiectasia and fibrosis following radiation treatment of tongue carcinoma.

they are included in the beam of radiation for most oral cancers. Therefore, patients will develop a partial (hypogeusia) or more usually, complete (ageusia) loss of taste during treatment. The alterations in taste for sweet, sour, bitter, and salt are variable and are caused by damage to the cells in the taste buds and/or their innervating nerve fibers. Often, some taste buds are altered, causing confusing perceptions of taste (dysgeusia). The cells comprising taste buds usually will regenerate within 4 months after treatment. However, the degree of long-term impairment of taste is quite variable from patient to patient.

Dietary consultations regarding recipes with pleasing texture and perceptible and pleasing tastes are essential to improve intake of food. However, there are tremendous patient-to-patient differences, which preclude standard recommendations. Failure in taste perception, in addition to pain, dysphagia, hyposalivation and depression, is associated with the loss of pleasure in eating, thus, a loss of appetite. This is compounded by frustrations in food preparation. Weight loss, weakness, malaise and dehydration often follow. This is further complicated when prior surgery has caused problems in mastication and swallowing. Trials with zinc supplements exceeding recommended daily doses appear to be helpful in some patients (100 mg elemental zinc daily). In addition to improving taste perception in some patients, zinc has occasionally improved saliva production. While zinc serves as a critical enzyme in many biochemical reactions, its role in taste and saliva remains unknown. Saliva probably has a modulating effect on the acuity of some tastes (sour, bitter, salt, sweet) through biochemical interactions, as well as providing an ionic environment in signal transduction for taste cells.

Salivary Function

Exposure of the major salivary glands to the field of ionizing radiation induces fibrosis, fatty degeneration, acinar atrophy, and cellular necrosis within glands. A critical dose level has not been identified. The serous acini appear to be more sensitive than the mucinous. During irradiation, the glandular secretions are usually diminished, thick, sticky, and very bothersome to the patient. Some patients are unable to produce more than 1 ml of pooled saliva in 10 min. The duration of this depressed salivary function varies from patient to patient. In most patients, there is usually some regeneration several months after treatment, and the undesirable signs and symptoms of xerostomia (discomfort, difficulty in speech and swallowing) are at least partially reversed. However, recovery of adequate saliva for oral comfort and function may take from 6 to 12 months; in others the saliva remains inadequate indefinitely and is the source of major posttreatment complaints. When both of the parotid glands are exposed to the treatment beam, saliva diminution is most marked, and the prognosis for recovery is the worst. Obviously, the higher the dosage of irradiation, the worse the prognosis for xerostomia.

Frequent sips of water and water rinses are essential for partial control of radiation-induced xerostomia. Sugarless chewing gum and tart candy may be helpful. In some patients, pilocarpine hydrochloride (solution or tablets) has been effective in stimulating saliva production [8]. Five milligrams 3–4 times daily has been an optimal dosage for most patients. Side effects can include sweating and stomach discomfort, but this usually occurs only at higher dosages.

In a double-blind controlled study of 12 patients irradiated for head and neck cancer at the Oral Medicine Clinic, University of California, San Francisco, pilocarpine administration (15–30 mg daily) appeared to be beneficial. All 12 patients had marked xerostomia which had failed to improve even though 6 months had elapsed since radiation treatment. After receiving pilocarpine, 9 of 12 improved subjectively, 9 of 12 had increased stimulated parotid flow rates, and 6 of 12 demonstrated improvement in whole saliva volume. While on placebo medication for 3 months, none of 12 showed objective or subjective benefit. Other studies have reported similar findings. Another salivary gland stimulant, bethanechol (Urecholine®), administered as tablets in divided doses varying from 75 to 200 mg daily, has been helpful in many xerostomic patients. However, it is not FDA-approved for this effect.

Synthetic saliva solutions and saliva substitute lubricants have been of limited help in the majority of patients with dry mouth, although some favorable reports have been published. In some patients in whom the salivary complaint is related to the 'thickness' (excess mucous-type secretions), guaifenesin (Organidin® NR) may help as a mucolytic agent (200–400 mg, 3–4 times daily).

Nutrition

Because of the painful mucositis, loss of taste, and partial xerostomia, the lack of desire or frank inability to eat is a common and almost universal complaint in patients receiving external irradiation to the oral cavity. This is particularly the case when the field includes the oropharynx. These changes, in combination with difficulty in mastication and swallowing caused by the tumor and the treatment, will result in weight loss. A marked weight loss tends to permit weakness, inactivity, discouragement, further anorexia, and susceptibility to infection. Therefore, close attention is given to food intake and weight maintenance during treatment and follow-up. Dietary supplements, menu preparations, and encouragement to eat become important factors. Diets vary, depending upon patient attitude and effort, previous surgical intervention, saliva and taste status, food texture, and pain.

There is usually very little change in the peripheral blood count before, during or after head and neck treatment, either in response to poorer nutrition or to irradiation. Therefore, anemia, bleeding, or immune deficiencies have not been complications.

Dental Caries

Patients who have not shown any degree of caries activity for years may develop dental decay and varying degrees of disintegration after irradiation (fig. 3A–C). The cervical areas are most typically affected. This condition appears to be due to the lack of saliva as well as to changes in its chemical composition. One result of radiation xerostomia is a pronounced shift toward a highly acidogenic, highly cariogenic oral microflora. The protective influence of saliva has been demonstrated by the extensive dental destruction found in animals subjected to salivary gland ligation or removal and in patients with xerostomia caused by drugs (e.g., diuretics, antidepressants) or disease (e.g., Sjögren's syndrome).

Radiation-induced dental effects primarily depend upon salivary changes, and occur when the glands are included in the field of treatment, not upon direct irradiation of the teeth themselves. Direct irradiation of teeth may alter the organic or inorganic components in some manner, making them more susceptible to decalcification; but this has not been shown clearly. Remineralization of enamel by a salivary substitute has been reported. There do not appear to be any clinical or histologic pulpal differences in noncarious human adult teeth, whether they have been in or out of the primary field of radiation. Studies in monkeys have also found no dental pulp damage.

To prevent or at least minimize radiation caries, oral hygiene must be maximal, including intensive home care and frequent office visits for exam-

---

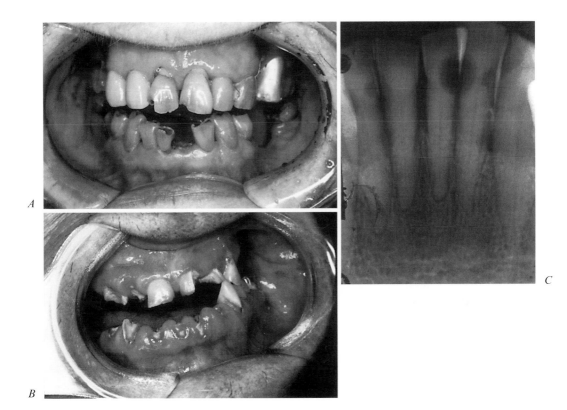

Fig. 3. A Radiation caries occurring 3 years after the completion of therapy. Note typical incisal and cervical caries. The crown of an incisor fractured off from the advanced carious decalcification. Patient compliance with oral hygiene and the use of topical fluorides was poor. *B* Severe dental destruction from 5 years of xerostomia following radiotherapy, poor oral hygiene, and nonuse of fluoride rinses or dentifrices. *C* Radiography of typical radiation-induced cervical caries.

ination and prophylaxis. Mouth rinsing is essential. Antiseptic mouth rinses, for example, chlorhexidine, if tolerated, are helpful in eliminating debris and controlling microbial flora. Daily topical fluoride applications, either as a solution for mouth rinsing, a gel delivered by means of a tray, or brushed on as a paste or gel, are all effective [9, 10]. Attempts should be made to increase salivary flow either by local or systemic means. Foods and beverages containing sucrose should be avoided as much as possible. If carious lesions develop, removal and restoration should take place immediately. Appropriate use of dental x-ray imaging is in order when indicated to monitor caries activity.

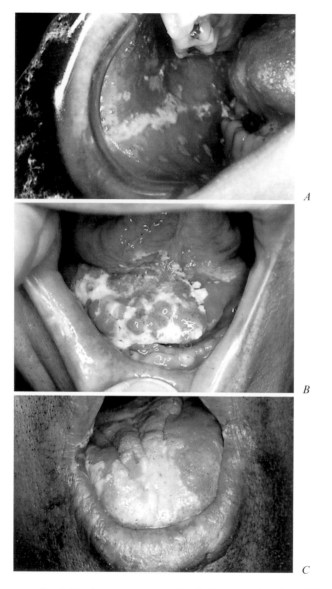

Fig. 4. Varying appearances of radiotherapy-induced candidiasis secondary to xerostomia. *A* Buccal mucosa. *B* Floor of mouth. *C* Tongue. Note the angular cheilitis and the confusing similarity to mucositis.

Table 1. Occurrence of oral *Candida* in 109 irradiated oral cancer patients[1]

Percent of patients	*Candida* culture		
	before therapy	end of therapy	after therapy[2]
41	Negative	Negative	Negative
10	Negative	Negative	Positive
27	Negative	Positive	Positive
22	Positive	Positive	Positive

[1] Data from Silverman et al., 1984 (67 men, 42 women).
[2] Mean time, 14 months.

Candidiasis

Infections of the mouth by *Candida albicans* are commonly seen in irradiated patients (fig. 4A–C, table 1), and are related to the alterations in saliva. Clinically the signs may be confused with radiation mucositis or other sources of infection. Candidiasis is usually painful. Management is primarily with the use of antifungal drugs. Systemic administration (200 mg ketoconazole daily with food, or fluconazole 100 mg daily) is usually more effective for both response and compliance. Duration of treatment depends upon control of signs and recurrences. Topical administration entails the use of nystatin or clotrimazole tablets dissolved orally. Because of pain from mucositis and dryness, patients may experience difficulty in dissolving tablets topically. Suspensions are another alternative form of treatment, but often this treatment is not as effective as the tablets (possibly because of limited contact time between drug and fungus). These fungal-control approaches are often used in combination. Antiseptic mouth rinses similar to those used for caries control may be helpful, if tolerated. In addition, topical (viscous xylocaine) or systemic analgetics may be required. Keeping the mouth moist is essential. There is always the possibility of developing fungal resistance, or the need of higher dosages, when these agents are used for prolonged periods of time.

Osteoradionecrosis

Osteonecrosis is one of the more serious complications of head and neck irradiation for cancer (fig. 5A, B). Bone cells and vascularity may be irreversibly injured (fig. 6A–C). Fortunately, in many cases devitalized bone fragments will sequestrate and lesions will spontaneously heal. However, when radiation osteonecrosis is progressive, it can lead to intolerable pain or fracture and may necessitate jaw resection. The preventive and therapeutic use of antibiotics

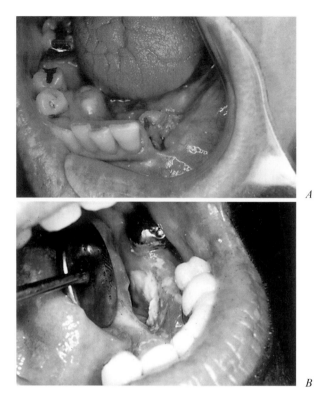

A

B

Fig. 5. A Osteonecrosis following a bicuspid extraction 3 years after the completion of radiotherapy for a tongue-floor of mouth carcinoma. The calculated bone dose exceeded 6,500 cGy. *B* Spontaneous mandibular osteonecrosis 2 years following external plus interstitial irradiation. Because of pain and extension, a segmental resection was required for control.

and hyperbaric oxygen can be effective, but reproducible beneficial results remain uncertain [11, 12].

The incidence of osteoradionecrosis varies depending upon the reporting institution, aggressiveness of radiotherapy, and follow-up time (table 2). The risk for developing spontaneous osteoradionecrosis is somewhat unpredictable, but it is related to the dose of radiation delivered and bone volume. The risk is increased in dentulous patients, even more if teeth within the treatment field are removed after therapy. Spontaneous bone exposure usually occurs more than 1 year after radiation is completed.

Animal models to study the effects of ionizing radiation on jaw bones have demonstrated changes similar to those observed in human specimens:

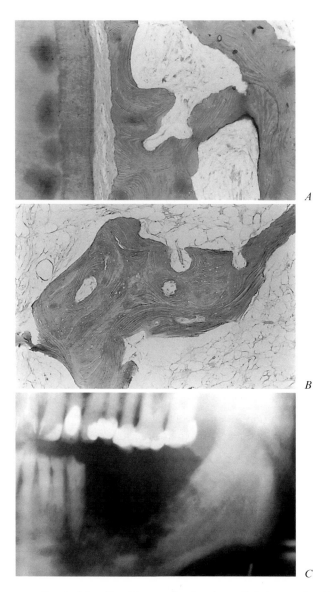

Fig. 6. A Irradiated bone reflecting the acellularity causing 'devitalized bone'. Left to right: dentin, cementum, periodontal ligament, alveolar bone. *B* A photomicrograph ($\times 400$) of bone trabecula showing no osteocytes, osteoblasts or osteoclasts and adjacent avascular marrow with fatty degeneration. *C* Radiograph of mandibular osteonecrosis. Continued expansion and pain required partial mandibulectomy.

Table 2. Reported incidence of osteonecrosis in patients irradiated for head and neck cancer

Source, Year	Hospital	Patients n	Years	Dosage cGy	Cases of osteonecrosis
Beumer, 1972	Univ. California (S.F.)	278	1961–69	5,000–7,000	10 (4%)
Bedwinek, 1976	M.D. Anderson (Tex.)	381	1966–71	6,000–7,500	54 (14%)
Murray, 1980	M.D. Anderson (Tex.)	397	1971–75	4,000–>8,000	77 (19%)
Morrish, 1981	Univ. California (S.F.)	100	1971–77	5,000–7,500	22 (22%)

Table 3. Incidence of osteonecrosis according to radiation dose to bone[1]

Dose to bone, cGy	Incidence of osteonecrosis	
	dentulous patients	edentulous patients
<6,500	0/36 (0%)	0/3 (0%)
6,500–7,500	8/29 (28%)	1/15 (7%)
>7,500	11/13 (85%)	2/4 (50%)
Total	19/78 (24%)	3/22 (14%)

[1] Data from Morrish et al., 1981.

marrow avascularity and fatty degeneration, reduction of osteocytes, osteoblasts and osteoclasts, enlarged lacunae, and microfractures.

University of California Study

To assess the contributory factors in the development of osteoradionecrosis, the records of 100 patients irradiated for head and neck cancer at the University of California, San Francisco, were reviewed retrospectively [13]. The group comprised 60 men and 40 women whose average age was 65 years. At the time of diagnosis, 78 were dentulous and 22 were edentulous. All patients received megavoltage external beam radiotherapy and/or interstitial radium or iridium implants. The maxilla and/or mandible were within the radiation fields. Special care was taken to calculate the bone dose as well as the tumor dose. The dose of external beam radiotherapy was in the range of 5,000–7,500 cGy, delivered at 180 cGy/fraction, five daily fractions per week. The total radiation dose included the dose from the external beam and from the interstitial implant (tables 3, 4).

Certain facts emerge from this study: (1) Patients who were edentulous at the time of diagnosis of cancer had a relatively low risk of osteonecrosis.

Table 4. Association of dental extractions and osteonecrosis in 78 irradiated dentulous patients[1]

Radiation dose, cGy			Osteonecrosis	
time or extraction	range	mean	incidence	mean time of onset after treatment, months
No extractions	6,940–9,280	7,871	5/41 (12%)	29
Before radiotherapy	7,580–9,610	8,500	3/19 (16%)	41
After radiotherapy	6,700–8,100	7,346	11/18 (61%)	20
Total	6,700–9,610	7,666	19/78 (24%)	22

[1] Data from Morrish et al., 1981. Radiation for dentulous patients without osteonecrosis ranged between 4,950 and 9,700 cGy (mean 6,450).

(2) Patients who were dentulous had a greater risk. (3) The increased risk in dentulous patients appeared to be associated with those who had tooth extractions after radiation therapy. (4) Dentulous patients with pretreatment extractions or no extractions appeared to have risks similar to those of the edentulous patients. (5) Spontaneous osteoradionecrosis can occur. (6) The most important risk factor for the development of osteonecrosis appeared to be the radiation dose to the bone, particularly in the mandible. (7) Clinical changes in skin and/or mucosa indicating radiation damage was a risk indicator for osteonecrosis. (8) The risk for osteonecrosis continues indefinitely following radiation therapy.

Treatment for Osteoradionecrosis

If osteonecrosis does not progress clinically or radiographically, the usual management involves periodic observation. If flares (swelling, suppuration, pain) occur only occasionally, antibiotics are usually effective. If pain and/or flares occur too frequently or present other difficulties for the patient, surgery must be considered.

Soft Tissue Necrosis

Soft tissue necrosis may be defined as the occurrence of a mucosal ulcer in irradiated tissue that has no residual cancer (fig. 7). The incidence of soft tissue necrosis is related to dose, time, and volume irradiated. The risk is far greater with interstitial implantation and intraoral techniques because of the higher irradiation doses used.

In a University of California, San Francisco, study of 278 patients, soft tissue necrosis occurred in 18 cases (6.5%). Eleven of these patients had been

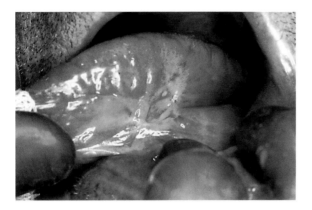

Fig. 7. Soft tissue necrosis occurring 14 months following the completion of external beam and interstitial irradiation for tongue carcinoma. There is often confusion between necrosis and recurrent tumor.

treated by needle implantation or intraoral cone techniques. The average time of onset was within a year of therapy. Fifteen cases were self-limiting, in time periods ranging from 1 to 10 months (average 3 months), but 3 cases required surgical intervention.

Soft tissue necrosis is usually quite painful. Optimal hygiene is required and analgetics are usually helpful, but antibiotics are generally of little help in relieving pain and promoting healing. Since these ulcerations are often at the site of the primary tumor, periodic assessment for recurrence is essential until the necrosis heals.

Dental Treatment Planning

In view of the risk that accompanies high-dose irradiation, special attention to preradiation dental planning appears critical. Factors important in the dental management of these patients include the following: (1) anticipated bone dose; (2) pretreatment dental status, dental hygiene, and retention of teeth that will be exposed to high-dose irradiation; (3) extraction techniques; (4) allowance of adequate healing time for teeth extracted before radiotherapy, and (5) patient motivation and capability of compliance to preventive measures.

Since many infections occur months or years after treatment, it is evident that the tissue changes induced by radiation persist for long periods of time and may be irreversible. Therefore, extreme care must be taken in evaluating the status of the teeth and periodontium before, during, and after treatment, and optimal oral and periodontal hygiene must be maintained because of the lowered biologic potential for healing in response to physical irritation, chemical agents, and microbial organisms. Such attention is critical because of the potentially progressive nature of radiation osteonecrosis, which may involve large segments of bone and present a major therapeutic problem, possibly requiring extensive resection.

It is impossible to establish precise formulas for managing preradiation and postradiation dental problems. Extractions are considered primarily for teeth with a poor prognosis due to conditions such as advanced periodontal disease, extensive caries, and periapical lesions. Other considerations are sources of chronic soft-tissue irritation (trauma), and the degree of patient cooperation in preventive home care and dental office programs. The decision is modified further for each patient on the basis of the individual's prognosis, age, desires, economic aspects, and radiation delivery.

Reported studies and personal experience do not substantiate the advisability of extracting all teeth before treatment as a good preventive measure. When teeth are extracted before or after irradiation, the alveolar bone must be evenly trimmed and carefully smoothed so that a primary tissue closure is possible. This is necessary because suppression of bone cell viability diminishes remodeling, and if a suitable alveolectomy is not performed, the resulting alveolar ridge will be irregular and may increase the risk of subsequent bone exposure and discomfort. A minimum of 1 week to 10 days is arbitrarily allowed for initial healing before radiation is instituted. However, if the situation permits, more time is preferable, up to 14 or even 21 days. Since dosages are fractionated, healing can usually continue before damaging levels of radiation are delivered to a surgical area. Obviously, teeth completely out of the treatment field are not affected to the same degree.

There is no evidence from studies as to how many teeth should be extracted at one time. Whether before or after irradiation, all of the teeth indicated for removal may be extracted as suits the surgeon's assessment of the needs of the patient. The use of antibiotics during the healing period is important to minimize infection. Whenever possible, an attempt is made to retain teeth to support tooth-borne applicances for the tentatively planned rehabilitation of these patients.

The periodontium is maintained in optimal condition by periodic routine periodontal procedures. When areas exposed to radiation are treated, extreme care is exercised and antibiotics may be selectively administered. Fluoride applications (daily, in the form of mouth rinses or gels) appear to aid in minimizing tooth decalcification and caries in these patients. There are no unusual contraindications for endodontic procedures.

In conclusion, review of the literature and our own experience indicate that carefully controlled studies are necessary before more definitive guidelines can be formulated for managing dental structures which have been or are to be irradiated. This is particularly true because of newer fractionation and dose regimens of radiation, as well as combinations with chemotherapy, in order to attain better responses and survival rates. Each case must be managed individually, based on the patient's needs, the status of the tumor, and the risks known to exist for dental health in irradiated tissues, and a one-formulae approach for all patients is contraindicated.

References

1   Cooper JS, Fu K, Marks J, Silverman S Jr: Late effects of radiation therapy in the head and neck region. Int J Radiat Oncol Biol Phys 1995;31:1141–1164.
2   List MA, D'Antonio LL, Cella DF, Siston A, Mumby P, Haraf D, Vokes E: The Performance Status Scale for Head and Neck Cancer Patients and the Functional Assessment of Cancer Therapy – Head and Neck Scale. A study of utility and validity. Cancer 1996;77:2295–2301.
3   Silverman S: Radiation and chemotherapy injury: Pathophysiology, diagnosis, and treatment. Crit Rev Oncol Hematol 1993;15:63–67.
4   Silverman S: Oral cavity toxicity secondary to chemotherapy and radiation therapy; in John M (ed): Chemoradiation. Philadelphia, Lea Febiger, 1993.
5   Rugg T, Saunders MI, Dische S: Smoking and mucosal reactions to radiotherapy. Br J Radiol 1990; 63:554–556.
6   Bruera E, Pereira J, Watanabe S, Belzile M, Kuehn N, Hanson J: Opioid rotation in patients with cancer pain. A retrospective comparison of dose ratios between methadone, hydromorphone, and morphine. Cancer 1996;78:852–857.
7   Levy MH: Pharmacologic treatment of cancer pain. N Engl J Med 1996;335:1124–1132.
8   Reike JW, Hafermann MD, Johnson JT, Le Veque FG: Oral pilocarpine for radiation-induced xerostomia: Integrated efficacy and safety results from two prospective randomized clinical trials. Int J Radiat Oncol Biol Phys 1995;31:661–669.
9   Epstein JB, van der Meij EH, Lunn R, Stevenson-Moore P: Effects of compliance with fluoride gel application on caries and caries risk in patients after radiation therapy for head and neck cancer. Oral Surg Oral Med Oral Pathol Oral Radiol Endod 1996;82:268–275.
10   Toljanic JA, Siddiqui AA, Patterson GL, Irwin ME: An evaluation of a dentifrice containing salivary peroxidase elements for the control of gingival disease in patients with irradiated head and neck cancer. J Prosth Dent 1996;76:292–296.
11   Van Merkesteyn JPR, Baker DJ, Borgmeijer-Hoelen AMMJ: Hyperbaric oxygen treatment of osteoradionecrosis of the mandible. Oral Surg Oral Med Oral Pathol Oral Radiol Endod 1995;80: 12–16.
12   Tibbles PM, Edelsberg JS: Hyperbaric-oxygen therapy. N Engl J Med 1996;335:1642–1648.
13   Morrish RB, Chan E, Silverman S Jr, Fu K: Osteonecrosis in patients irradiated for head and neck carcinoma. Cancer 1981;47:1980.

Dr. Sol Silverman, Jr., School of Dentistry, Box 0422,
University of California, San Francisco, CA 94143 (USA)
Tel. +1 415 476 5947, Fax +1 415 476 4204

Meyer JL (ed): Radiation Injury. Advances in Management and Prevention.
Front Radiat Ther Oncol. Basel, Karger, 1999, vol 32, pp 49–62

········ ··· ··· ········

Surgical Management of Radiation-Injured Tissues of the Head and Neck

Mike Yao, David J. Terris

Division of Otolaryngology/Head and Neck Surgery, Stanford University Medical
Center, Stanford, Calif., USA

Most advanced stage head and neck cancers are treated with combined
therapy consisting of surgery and radiotherapy. Modern techniques using
multiple radiation ports and fractionation have increased the safety and efficacy
of radiotherapy, and are designed to maximize killing of tumor cells while
minimizing damage to normal tissues. Complications of treatment do occur,
however. In the head and neck, the problem of radiation damage is particularly
challenging because of the complex anatomy and proximity of the soft tissues
to the underlying bony architecture. In this review, we will focus on the nonsurgical and surgical management of specific complications that arise from irradiation of head and neck neoplasms, utilizing illustrative case examples.

Acute and Chronic Effects of Radiation

Two phases of radiation injury are recognized: acute (occurring during
the first 6 months) and chronic (developing more than 6 months after radiation). Acute injuries result from the reproductive death of rapidly dividing
cells, due to DNA damage. Some acute injuries will heal over time because
of a transition of the remaining stem cells into a state of accelerated repopulation. After severe radiation injuries, the entire stem cell population may be
destroyed, preventing recovery from the acute injury. Chronic injuries are
caused by radiation damage to the slowly dividing parenchymal cells and the
microvasculature.

Clinically, acute radiation injuries are manifested as mucositis, dermatitis,
xerostomia and ageusia, stemming from the radiosensitivity of epithelial tissues, serous salivary glands, and taste buds, respectively. These normal tissue

effects will result if a comprehensive curative course of radiotherapy is undertaken for a head and neck malignancy [1]. Modern radiation techniques help to minimize these acute injuries, and render them amenable to conservative medical therapy.

Chronic radiation injuries are manifested as osteoradionecrosis, dental disease, fistulae, tissue necrosis, fibrosis, and carotid exposure/injury. These changes may progress even after radiation has been completed because of continued cell death. These injuries are generally more severe than the acute injuries. Conservative medical management is not always effective, and surgical intervention is needed at times. Because these injuries reflect radiotherapy technique, prevention is one of the principal forms of management of chronic radiation injury.

Radiation Injuries Requiring Nonsurgical Management

Mucositis

The rapidly proliferating basal cells of the mucosal epithelium are exquisitely sensitive to radiation. Two to 3 weeks (20–30 Gy) after the initiation of a course of head and neck radiation, enough of these basal cells are killed to cause superficial mucosal ulcerations referred to as mucositis [1]. The main objective in therapy of this condition is to minimize the pain so that it does not interfere with adequate nutritional intake, which is known to be important for proper wound healing.

Patients should avoid irritants such as alcohol and tobacco, and rinse frequently with saline soda solutions to decrease painful mucosal irritation. Local anesthetic mouthwashes and narcotic analgesics are often indicated. In cases of superinfection with *Candida*, nystatin oral rinses or clotrimazole troches are usually curative. Systemic therapy with fluconazole may become necessary. If eating becomes too painful for the patient to maintain his weight, then nutritional support with nasogastric feeding or parenteral hyperalimentation should be initiated.

Occasionally, in very severe cases of mucositis causing edema of the upper airway, intubation or tracheotomy is necessary. Temporary cessation of radiation may be needed to treat these complications. The mucosal epithelium will usually grow back within about 2 weeks following a curative course of radiation (60–70 Gy) [1].

Dermatitis

Radiation skin injury begins with erythema in the radiation field and may progress to dry desquamation, then to moist desquamation and finally frank ulceration. The erythematous reaction occurs approximately 8 days after a single dose of 800 cGy and reaches its peak 8 days later. This erythema is thought to be due to an inflammatory reaction to damage of the basal cell population in the epidermis. Dry desquamation occurs when an intermediate dose of radiation kills some of the epidermal cells, but enough survive to repopulate the skin within 1 month. Like mucositis, wet desquamation occurs when radiation kills virtually all the basal cells within a treatment field and the dermis is exposed. Ulceration occurs when areas of wet desquamation are so damaged that they are not capable of any type of repair.

Treatment of radiation-damaged skin consists mostly of supportive measures. Traumatic and irritative activities such as shaving, scratching, sun exposure, and the application of alcohol-based emollients or cosmetics should be avoided. Topical moisturizers, such as *Aloe vera* and Vigilon provide moderate relief.

Wet desquamation may require temporary cessation of radiation therapy. The application of clean, wet-to-dry saline dressings 3–4 times a day will mechanically debride the wound. Following debridement, antibiotic ointments and creams, such as silver sulfadiazine, can reduce bacterial colonization and facilitate re-epithelialization.

Even with appropriate management, some wounds will continue to enlarge. Since large, nonhealing wounds may represent a tumor recurrence, malignancy must be ruled out. Nonhealing wounds require excision of the central ulcers as well as the surrounding abnormal tissue [2]. Following excision, the wounds heal best when covered with vascularized tissue from outside the radiation field.

Xerostomia

Xerostomia is an unavoidable side effect of curative courses of radiotherapy. When the salivary glands receive >50 Gy of irradiation, xerostomia can be severe and to a degree permanent [3], causing difficult deglutition and predisposing to caries.

Sialagogues and salivary substitutes are the most commonly used agents for symptomatic relief. Pilocarpine, a muscarinic cholinergic agonist, may be prescribed to stimulate any remaining functional salivary gland tissue, improving salivary flow and subjective symptoms. When no salivary function remains, carboxymethylcellulose-based saliva substitutes are the mainstay of therapy in the United States. In Europe, mucin-based saliva substitutes are available [3].

Radiation Injuries Requiring Surgical Management

Osteoradionecrosis

Pathophysiology

The necrotizing effects of radiation on bone were recognized as early as 1926 [4]. This condition, known as osteoradionecrosis (ORN), was originally thought to consist of the triad of radiation, trauma and infection. However, Marx [5] in 1983 was only able to culture organisms from the surface of 12 mandibles resected for ORN. Since all deep cultures were negative, he concluded that microorganisms play a minor role in the pathophysiology of ORN of the mandible.

In his description of the pathophysiology of ORN, Marx [5] cited the lethal effects of radiation on the cells within the mandible such as osteocytes and osteoblasts, which result in hypocellular bone. The effects of radiation on the microvasculature also cause hypovascularity, and ultimately leading to tissues that are hypoxic relative to unirradiated tissues. These '3 Hs' (hypocellularity, hypovascularity and hypoxia) cause tissues to lose their ability to initiate normal repair. This compromised tissue is then either susceptible to spontaneous breakdown or is unable to repair insults in a timely fashion. The clinical course of radiation tissue injury over time is shown in figure 1. At the completion of radiation therapy, patients are vulnerable to trauma-induced ORN. However, during the 6 months immediately following the completion of radiation, the risk of ORN is low because the natural repair processes heal the acute radiation injury. This risk subsequently increases as a result of the late effects of radiation, such as late mitotic death, increasing fibrosis and microvascular damage. The gradual accumulation of postradiation damage in some cases will progress to spontaneous ORN. The risk for ORN continues to increase for at least 7 years following the completion of radiation, and precipitating factors include infection, surgery and trauma.

The mandible is particularly susceptible to ORN because of the mechanical stress of chewing, which may cause microfractures. In a normal metabolic state, this bone heals itself without difficulty, but in the compromised postradiation state, the bone cannot heal the fractures quickly enough to avoid the compounding of several microfractures together, eventually resulting in a pathologic fracture. The risk of ORN is correlated with radiation dose [6–9], fractionation dose [8], tumor size [6], and bony involvement by the tumor [9, 10].

Dental disease has been identified as a major cause of ORN. A preradiation dental evaluation is essential, as the rate of ORN in patients who undergo postirradiation extraction is much higher than in those who have preirradiation extraction. If the radiographs and physical examination reveal healthy dentition, the risk for ORN is low [11], and prophylactic extraction is not advised.

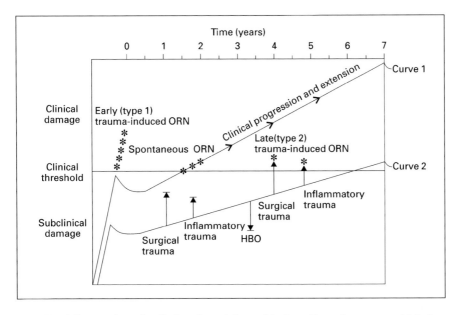

Fig. 1. Progression of radiation tissue injury with time. Curve 1 represents high-dose radiation with a goal of killing as many tumor cells as possible while avoiding ORN (as represented by the clinical threshold line). Curve 1 crosses the clinical threshold line at two points, representing two of the ORN groups. The first, the early trauma-induced ORN depicted by extension of the therapy line in asterisks, shows that at the completion of radiation patients are vulnerable to trauma, such as surgical intervention. The second, the spontaneous ORN depicted by the asterisks on the gradually sloping line, shows that the gradual accumulation of postradiation damage in some cases will progress to spontaneous ORN. Curve 2 represents radiation tissue injury well below the clinical threshold for ORN. The long-term upward slope shows that the risk for ORN continues to increase for at least 7 years following the completion of radiation. The upward vertical arrows represent insults, such as infections or surgery, which can in some cases precipitate ORN, resulting in the late, trauma-induced group of ORN patients. The effect of hyperbaric oxygen therapy can be seen as a downward pointing arrow that moves the curve away from the clinical threshold. (Reprinted with permission from Marx and Johnson [8].)

Manifestations/Evaluation

The diagnosis of ORN requires a wound with exposed, irradiated bone that has failed to heal over a period of 3 months [12]. ORN can occur in the maxilla and temporal bone, but it is most commonly seen in the mandible. The reported incidence of ORN of the mandible following radiation ranges from 2.6 to 22% [6, 13]. The most frequent complaint associated with ORN of the mandible is pain [10]. Other symptoms that may be seen in conjunction with ORN are hypesthesia, dysesthesia, odor, dysgeusia and trismus. Untreated ORN may lead to pathologic fractures, fistulae and systemic infection.

The panorex is the most cost-effective radiographic study for evaluating ORN [12] and may be used to identify pathologic fractures, or sequestrum formation which can be seen as irregular areas of opacification within areas of radiolucency. Panorex findings may not reflect the true extent of the disease, however, and consideration should be given to obtaining a CT scan or Denta-scan. These studies are especially useful for the detection of soft tissue masses in the region of bone resorption which may represent recurrent cancer. The erythrocyte sedimentation rate (ESR) may be used as a harbinger of possible osteomyelitis, and in cases when the ESR is elevated, a falling ESR may act as an indication of successful therapy [12]. Since all of the findings of ORN are consistent with recurrent or metastatic carcinoma, biopsies to rule out carcinoma must be performed prior to any therapy, when ORN occurs near the original tumor site.

Treatment

The management of ORN begins with conservative measures such as avoidance of mucosal irritants (alcohol, tobacco, dentures), the use of saline irrigation, oral antibiotics when infection is present, topical antiseptics and antibiotic packing, and gentle debridement, including sequestrectomies when necessary. Between 70 and 97% of patients will heal or stabilize their wounds with these conservative measures [6, 7]. Hyperbaric oxygen has proven to be beneficial in the treatment of ORN. The transient elevations in tissue oxygen tension provided by the HBO dives stimulate collagen synthesis and fibroblast proliferation, ultimately inducing angiogenesis and neocellularity of the osteo-radionecrotic wound [14]. The tissue vascularity increases to a plateau at 80–85% of the vascularity of nonirradiated tissue by 20 dives [15]. This in-creased vascularity has the long-term effect of reducing the risk of spontaneous or trauma-induced ORN [8], but HBO without aggressive surgical manage-ment will not resolve the disease process in most instances [14].

Surgical intervention should be considered when nonsurgical measures fail, or in the event of intractable pain, orocutaneous fistula, persistent bone exposure or pathologic fracture. The basic principle of surgical management of ORN is resection of necrotic and heavily scarred tissue, and replacement with nonirradiated vascularized tissue [16]. Every effort should be made to preserve the continuity of the mandible.

Marx [14] has proposed a three-stage treatment protocol which combines the use of HBO and surgery for refractory ORN. In stage I, the patient is treated with HBO. If no improvement is noted on clinical examination, the patient proceeds to stage II, which consists of a transoral alveolar sequestrec-tomy with primary mucosal closure, and continued HBO therapy. In the event of dehiscence, resection of the mandible is performed after pretreatment with

HBO (stage III). Ten weeks after the resection, patients are given additional HBO therapy in preparation for bone graft reconstruction. All 58 patients treated under this protocol achieved resolution of their disease; 41 patients required stage III management (mandibular resection) [14].

Reconstruction

Reconstruction of mandibular defects after resection for ORN is generally undertaken after a delay of 3–6 months to ensure the absence of infection. While the three-dimensional reconstruction of complex bony defects is challenging and includes numerous options, some general principles and overall objectives should be understood. Both function and cosmesis must be addressed when reconstructing segmental mandibular defects. Some small lateral segmental defects can be left unreconstructed, without significant functional or cosmetic consequences. The four general approaches to mandibular defects, therefore, include conservative nonsurgical therapy, the use of metal reconstruction plates, implantation of nonvascularized corticocancellous particulate bone grafts, and vascularized osseous transfers.

While metal reconstruction plates have been used in ablative oncologic surgery for long-term mandibular continuity, they are generally used only for temporary reconstruction in patients with successfully treated disease. The advantages of reconstruction plates include the short operative time required, lack of donor site morbidity, capacity for precise molding of the plate (yielding superior cosmesis and anatomical alignment), avoidance of maxillomandibular fixation (which would otherwise impair the assessment of oral cavity healing), and improved ability to commence swallowing therapy [17]. The most significant drawback of plate reconstruction is the high rate of plate exposure in patients who have received radiation. In a prospective study, Klotch et al. [18] reported a 39% rate of plate exposure (intraoral, extraoral, or both) or fistula formation.

Nonvascularized corticocancellous particulate bone grafts have been used to reconstruct postresection defects in patients with ORN, but should be combined with adjuvant HBO. Marx and Ames [19] reported a 92% success rate when bone grafts were placed in irradiated beds which had been pretreated with HBO, which is thought to promote successful healing by improving the vascularity of the soft tissue envelope and neighboring host bone, thereby increasing the likelihood of revascularization of the graft. This compares with a 50% success rate in the absence of HBO. This revascularization is critical for maintenance of the size and function of the bone graft over time, and can also be achieved by transferring vascularized flaps to the recipient bed before bone grafting [16].

Vascularized osseus flaps may be pedicled or may require microvascular transfer. Pedicled flaps may be derived from local or distant tissues, but they maintain their original blood supply. Microvascular free bone flaps and their vascular pedicles are harvested from a distant site, and then the blood vessels are anastomosed to recipient bed vessels during the reconstruction. Both of these options allow for reconstruction with vascularized soft tissue and bone, with the potential for improving the viability of tissues in the recipient tissue bed.

A variety of pedicled composite flaps have been described, including the trapezius osteomyocutaneous flap, pectoralis osteomyocutaneous flap and the sternocleidomastoid flap (using a portion of the medial clavicle) [10, 20]. The osseus components of these flaps rely on the muscle to provide blood supply via periosteal perforators. This form of blood supply is not as robust as that from microvascular free flaps, and results in higher rates of nonunions, late bone resorption, and occasionally total necrosis of the bone.

Microvascular free flap transfer is currently the method of choice for reconstructing bony defects after resection of ORN [10]. Many sources of tissue for microvascular transfer have been described including the fibula, iliac crest, scapula, radius, rib, and metatarsal [10, 21]. The disadvantages of microvascular free flap reconstruction are increased operative time, high cost, and potential donor site morbidity.

Case 1: V.P. is a 57-year-old female with $T_2N_1M_0$ high-grade mucoepidermoid cancer of the left oral tongue first diagnosed in 1983. She was treated with a left partial glossectomy and left neck dissection, and postoperative radiation totalling 55 Gy to the left tongue and bilateral necks in 2.0-Gy fractions. She did well until May of 1991, when she manifested signs of ORN, and ultimately developed multiple orocutaneous fistulae (fig. 2). She was managed initially with antibiotics and local wound care. When the ORN persisted, she underwent HBO therapy (40 dives) without resolution of the fistulae or ORN. Advanced hip osteoarthritis led to the need for hip replacement in 1994 and because her orthopedic surgeons refused to operate while she still had the orocutaneous fistulae, surgical management of the ORN was advised. The patient underwent multiple fistulectomies, mandibular debridement, and local skin and mucosal flaps in March of 1994, with successful resolution of the ORN, allowing a hip replacement to be done later that year.

The principles of a staged approach to the management of ORN are illustrated in this patient, who failed conservative treatment with local wound care and antibiotics, proceeded to HBO therapy, and finally, was successfully managed with surgical resection of the ORN, while maintaining the continuity of the mandible.

Case 2: E.L. is a 67-year-old male with a left alveolar ridge SCCA first diagnosed in 1968. After failing radiation therapy totalling 70 Gy, he underwent curative resection consisting of a left composite resection. He did well for 20 years, but presented again in February of 1991 with right oral pain and x-rays suggestive of ORN (fig. 3). A biopsy was obtained, and revealed squamous cell carcinoma (SCCA). He was therefore treated with a right composite resection, and on routine examination in December of 1996 was noted to be without evidence of disease.

This case emphasizes the importance of vigilant cancer surveillance. Many of the symptoms and findings of ORN may also be seen in patients with recurrent cancer.

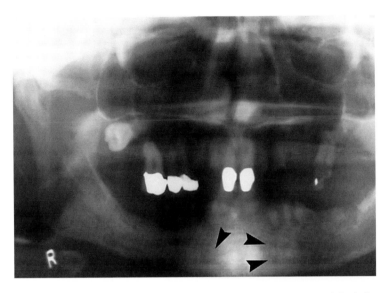

Fig. 2. Multiple orocutaneous fistulae with corresponding radiologic bony defects (see arrows) following left partial glossectomy and left neck dissection, and postoperative radiation.

Fistula

The incidence of fistula formation increases with the total radiation dose [22], and pharyngocutaneous fistula rates in some clinical situations may be as high as 31–34% [23]. Fistulae that develop in patients undergoing salvage surgery following curative courses of radiation are associated with the highest risk of carotid artery rupture [22]. Surgery following 50 Gy of radiation is associated with lower complication rates than for surgery following doses >65 Gy [23].

Treatment of fistulae begins with diversion of salivary flow to prevent continued contamination of the wound and/or carotid artery. This may be accomplished by mechanical techniques (packing or bypass tubes) or pharmacologic measures (glycopyrrolate to diminish secretions). Nasogastric feedings help to decrease flow through the fistula and provide important nutritional support for healing of the wound. Local wound care and debridement (either surgical or chemical, with hydrogen peroxide or Dakin's solution) are required to remove necrotic tissue and promote proper wound healing. Antibiotics are routinely used to minimize the bacterial count in secretions soiling the neck. Small fistulae usually close spontaneously with conservative measures. Larger fistulae may require vascularized (either pedicled or microvascular) flaps for closure.

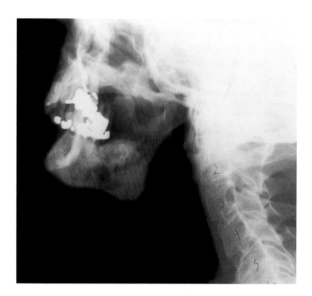

Fig. 3. Panorex showing the characteristic moth-eaten appearance, which was suggestive of ORN, but was proven to be squamous cell carcinoma.

The most feared consequence of a pharyngocutaneous fistula is carotid artery rupture. Bacterial and salivary enzymatic contamination can lead rapidly to necrosis and rupture of the arterial wall. A 'sentinel' or 'herald' bleed is a brief episode of hemorrhage which represents an impending carotid artery rupture. Control of bleeding may require ligation of the external, internal or common carotid arteries. Neurologic sequelae are best avoided by ensuring the patient is euvolemic and normotensive prior to ligation to optimize the conditions for cerebral perfusion. These wounds require immediate closure and coverage with vascularized flaps from outside the radiation field.

When they occur prior to postoperative adjuvant radiation, fistulae should be stabilized and the carotid artery protected, so that the radiation may be delivered as planned even if the fistula persists. Definitive closure of the fistula can be performed after the postradiation inflammation has resolved.

Tissue Necrosis/Flap Loss

Increasing doses of radiation produce incremental delays in wound healing [1]. Fibroblast depletion and microvascular damage (causing hypoxia) impair the reparative ability of the tissues. After resections for salvage of radiation failures, the surgical insult may overwhelm the healing capacity of the tissues, leading to frank tissue necrosis, and occasionally flap loss. Again, carotid artery rupture is the most feared consequence. As with fistulae, management of tissue necrosis begins with local wound care, which will promote the spontaneous resolution of many small areas of necrosis. Larger necrotic areas or flap losses require vascularized flaps for closure.

Case 3: L.M. is a 59-year-old male with a $T_4N_{2c}M_0$ SCCA of the left tonsil. He was treated in March of 1996 with neoadjuvant induction chemotherapy (cisplatin and 5-FU) and simultaneous chemoradiation. When his radiation dose had reached 22 Gy, he was determined to have progression of his disease. He therefore underwent surgical salvage with a left composite resection in July of 1996, and then received postoperative radiation consisting of an additional 38 Gy to the primary site and 28 Gy to the neck in 2.0-Gy fractions in August of 1996. During this postoperative radiation, he developed a left neck wound dehiscence. Local wound care was instituted, but the wound failed to heal, and in fact deteriorated into frank tissue necrosis (fig. 4a). He subsequently underwent a wide resection of necrotic tissue 2 months later, and the pathology confirmed widespread tissue necrosis. The wound then began healing rapidly, with granulation tissue appearing (fig. 4b). A split thickness skin graft was placed to hasten epithelialization, and the wound healed completely (fig. 4c).

Although most open wounds close spontaneously with local measures, this case provides an example of how necrotic tissue impairs wound healing and must therefore be widely resected on occasion. Delayed closure is preferred because high bacterial counts may prevent successful grafting when performed primarily.

Case 4: J.G. is a 64-year-old male with a $T_4N_0M_0$ SCCA of the left base of tongue and tonsil. He was diagnosed in July of 1993 (fig. 5a), and initially was treated with neoadjuvant induction chemotherapy and simultaneous chemoradiation with a total radiation dose of 70 Gy to the primary site and 50 Gy to the neck in 2.0-Gy fractions. Four months after the completion of therapy, he presented with a left tonsillar ulcer (fig. 5b), pain and a sentinel oropharyngeal bleed. He was taken urgently to the operating room for a wide resection of necrotic tissue, ligation of the external carotid artery and isolation of the internal carotid artery. A pectoralis major myocutaneous flap was used to replace the tissue deficit, and protect the carotid artery (fig. 5c). He is currently 3 years after treatment, has a well-healed oropharynx, and has no evidence of disease.

This final case represents a newer trend in the management of advanced head and neck cancers, the so-called 'organ preservation' protocols. These new protocols may bring with them a return to more surgical salvage of irradiated tissues and, as in the present example, reconstructive techniques to repair deficits created by tumor ulceration and necrosis. The importance of protecting the carotid arteries is re-emphasized.

In summary, radiation is a critical component in the treatment of early and advanced head and neck cancers. The acute side effects of mucositis, dermatitis, xerostomia and ageusia are unavoidable when a comprehensive, curative course of radiation is delivered. Fortunately, these complications can be managed with conservative measures and many resolve following cessation of the radiation.

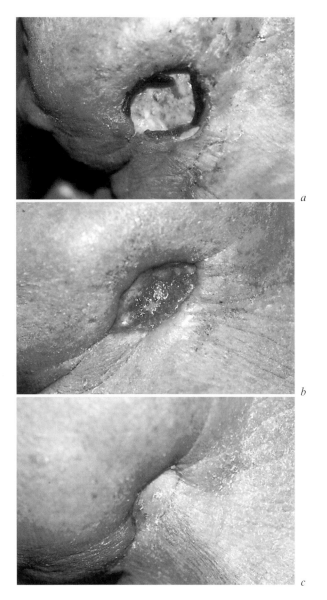

Fig. 4. a Tissue necrosis following wound dehiscence and failure of local wound care in a patient treated with induction chemotherapy and simultaneous chemoradiation, salvage surgery with left composite resection, and postoperative radiation. *b* Wound following wide resection of necrotic tissue showing rapid healing and granulation tissue. *c* Healed wound following split thickness skin graft.

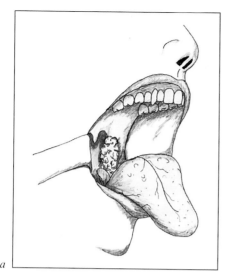

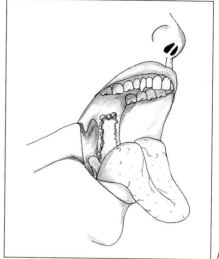

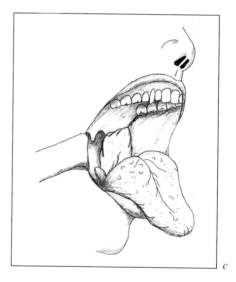

Fig. 5. a Large left tonsil and lateral
pharyngeal wall squamous cell carcinoma.
b Appearance of ulcer in the site of the previous cancer after treatment with an organ-
sparing protocol (cisplatin and 5-FU followed by simultaneous chemoradiation). The
patient presented at this point with a 'sentinel' bleed, and a ruptured external carotid
artery. c Postoperative appearance after ligation of the external carotid artery, and reconstruction of the defect with a pectoralis major
myocutaneous flap.

ORN, fistulae, and tissue necrosis may occur despite careful treatment
planning and gentle tissue handling. While medical therapy usually is sufficient
to manage these problems, surgical intervention is occasionally required. The
surgical principles that should be observed include aggressive removal of all
necrotic tissue and restoration of deficits with nonirradiated, vascularized flaps
when appropriate. Many reconstructive options are now available for these
tissue defects, with microvascular free flaps the treatment of choice in selected
situations.

References

1 Moore MJ: The effect of radiation on connective tissue. Otolaryngol Clin North Am 1984;17: 389–399.
2 Coleman JJD: Management of radiation-induced soft-tissue injury to the head and neck. Clin Plast Surg 1993;20:491–505.
3 Jacob RF: Management of xerostomia in the irradiated patient. Clin Plast Surg 1993;20:507–516.
4 Phemister D: Radium necrosis of bone. AJR 1926;16:340.
5 Marx RE: Osteoradionecrosis: A new concept of its pathophysiology. J Oral Maxillofac Surg 1983; 41:283–288.
6 Bedwinek JM, Shukovsky LJ, Fletcher GH, Daley TE: Osteonecrosis in patients treated with definitive radiotherapy for squamous cell carcinomas of the oral cavity and naso- and oropharynx. Radiology 1976;119:665–667.
7 Morrish RB Jr, Chan E, Silverman S Jr, Meyer J, Fu KK, Greenspan D: Osteonecrosis in patients irradiated for head and neck carcinoma. Cancer 1981;47:1980–1983.
8 Marx RE, Johnson RP: Studies in the radiobiology of osteoradionecrosis and their clinical significance. Oral Surg Oral Med Oral Pathol 1987;64:379–390.
9 Schratter-Sehn AU, Handl-Zeller L, Strassl H, Braun OM, Dobrowsky W: Incidence of osteoradionecrosis after combined radiotherapy-chemotherapy of head and neck tumors. Strahlenther Onkol 1991;167:165–168.
10 Sanger JR, Matloub HS, Yousif NJ, Larson DL: Management of osteoradionecrosis of the mandible. Clin Plast Surg 1993;20:517–530.
11 Murray CG, Daly TE, Zimmerman SO: The relationship between dental disease and radiation necrosis of the mandible. Oral Surg Oral Med Oral Pathol 1980;49:99–104.
12 Costantino PD, Friedman CD, Steinberg MJ: Irradiated bone and its management. Otolaryngol Clin North Am 1995;28:1021–1038.
13 Epstein JB, Rea G, Wong FL, Spinelli J, Stevenson-Moore P: Osteonecrosis: Study of the relationship of dental extractions in patients receiving radiotherapy. Head Neck Surg 1987;10:48–54.
14 Marx RE: A new concept in the treatment of osteoradionecrosis. J Oral Maxillofac Surg 1983;41: 351–357.
15 Marx RE, Johnson RP, Kline SN: Prevention of osteoradionecrosis: A randomized prospective clinical trial of hyperbaric oxygen versus penicillin. J Am Dent Assoc 1985;111:49–54.
16 Baker SR: Management of osteoradionecrosis of the mandible with myocutaneous flaps. J Surg Oncol 1983;24:282–289.
17 Saunders JR Jr, Hirata RM, Jaques DA: Definitive mandibular replacement using reconstruction plates. Am J Surg 1990;160:387–389.
18 Klotch DW, Gump J, Kuhn L: Reconstruction of mandibular defects in irradiated patients. Am J Surg 1990;160:396–398.
19 Marx RE, Ames JR: The use of hyperbaric oxygen therapy in bony reconstruction of the irradiated and tissue-deficient patient. J Oral Maxillofac Surg 1982;40:412–420.
20 Cuono CB, Ariyan S: Immediate reconstruction of a composite mandibular defect with a regional osteomusculocutaneous flap. Plast Reconstr Surg 1980;65:477–484.
21 Coleman JJD, Wooden WA: Mandibular reconstruction with composite microvascular tissue transfer. Am J Surg 1990;160:390–395.
22 Hom DB, Adams GL, Monyak D: Irradiated soft tissue and its management. Otolaryngol Clin North Am 1995;28:1003–1019.
23 Newman JP, Terris DJ, Pinto HA, Fee WE, Goode RL, Goffinet DR: Surgical morbidity of neck dissection after chemoradiotherapy in advanced head and neck cancer. Ann Otol Rhinol Laryngol 1997;106:117–122.

David J. Terris, MD, Division of Otolaryngology/Head and Neck Surgery,
R-135, Edwards Building, Stanford University Medical Center, Stanford, CA 94305-5328 (USA)
Tel. +1 650 725 6500, Fax +1 650 725 8502

Meyer JL (ed): Radiation Injury. Advances in Management and Prevention.
Front Radiat Ther Oncol. Basel, Karger, 1999, vol 32, pp 63–70

....

Lung Toxicity in the Treatment of Lung Cancer: Thoughts at the End of the Millennium

Charles R. Thomas, Jr., Todd E. Williams, Andrew T. Turrisi, III

Department of Radiation Oncology, Medical University of South Carolina,
Charleston, S.C., USA

The problem of lung cancer and its high mortality warrant the attention of clinical investigators in order to improve treatment and survival. As the tobacco epidemic continues, the mortality of lung cancer remains at the top of the list for the cancer problem throughout the world. Although there is rekindled interest in surgical therapy for patients with proven nodal disease and promising new, active chemotherapy agents, many patients are medically unfit for surgery or chemotherapy.

For most patients thoracic radiotherapy remains the mainstay of treating advanced local disease, or provides symptomatic relief from distant metastatic sites. The pillars of definitive radiotherapy for locally advanced disease have included a 'wide-field' approach, encompassing the clinical target, normal tissue margins, and regional lymph nodes. The normal tissue in the treated volume and its sensitivity have limited the total dose of radiotherapy. Unfortunately this has led to the use of a less than effective dose, only 60–65 Gy, which controls less than 10% of local tumors [Arriagada et al., 1997]. A concern about the consequences of radiation myelopathy has led to techniques that tend to expose more volume of lung to higher doses. As more effective chemotherapy is incorporated with local radiotherapy, toxic interactions to the lung and esophagus have limited the general use of these techniques, and possibly has interfered with the optimal methods of combining the modalities. Similarly, wide-field radiotherapy may also make its use as a partner with surgery, either preoperatively or postoperatively, more hazardous.

This chapter intends to probe the available information about lung toxicity, its mechanisms, and propose ways to prioritize risk more rationally in the treatment of lung cancer – *the larger risk of toxicity is to lung and esophagus rather than to the spinal cord.* Also, we need to re-evaluate the value, if any, of elective treatment of uninvolved nodal sites (hila, mediastinum, and supraclavicular fossae). We should assess the gain versus the risks that nodal treatment causes, both in limiting total doses and in exposing the lungs and esophagus to toxicity, either with radiotherapy alone, or with chemotherapy. Very likely, the amount of reserve functional lung capacity will limit radiotherapy, as it limits surgery. Consequently, new models are necessary and we shall need to move away from time-honored practices, whose value has not been proven but still continued based on appealing theory or analogy to other neoplastic processes.

Treatment-Related Lung Damage

Exposure of normal lung to ionizing radiation has had two well-recognized adverse sequelae: pneumonitis and pulmonary fibrosis [Mosvas et al., 1997]. Pneumonitis has been characterized by typical clinical and radiographic findings consisting of fever, dry cough and chest x-ray abnormalities that conventionally conform to the shape of the treatment port. Moreover, it is a diagnosis of exclusion: infection, lymphangitic spread, shock-lung, congestive heart failure, pulmonary embolism and hypersensitivity, all must be ruled out. Clinical pneumonitis occurs in about 10% of cases treated for lung cancer and occurs typically 4–6 weeks after completion of thoracic radiotherapy, perhaps earlier after combined chemoradiotherapy. Treatment factors related to pneumonitis are unclear, but dose, volume, fractionation have all been implicated [Rubin and Casarett, 1968; Roach et al., 1995; Mosvas et al., 1997; Byhardt et al., 1993].

The observed delay from completion of therapy until the clinical manifestation of pneumonitis has often been referred to as the 'latency period'. Current models dispel the idea that there is a period of quiescence, but rather an immediate active, subclinical cascade of molecular events that are initiated at the time of insult [Rubin et al., 1992; Finkelstein et al. 1994; Rodemann and Bamberg, 1995].

Pulmonary alveolar cells, lymphocytes and macrophages have a very complex interaction. After irradiation, there appears to be injury, reactive cells and a cascade of cytokines [King et al., 1989; Rubin et al., 1992; Finkelstein et al., 1994]. The target cells of injury appear to be the type II pneumocytes found in the alveolus and the alveolar capillary endothelial cells [Phillips, 1966; Finkelstein et al., 1994]. The interstitium between alveoli appear edematous, but remains free of cells. One of the normal functions of alveolar cells is the production of surfactant, the substance that allows the alveolus to remain open with less pressure. After irradiation, the type II cells immediately express injury by release of surfactant or pre-surfactant precursor. The type II cells are influenced by both transforming growth factors alpha (TGF-α) and beta (TGF-β) [Rubin et al., 1995]. The vascular endothelial cells is essential in gas exchange. When injured, these produce angiotensin-converting enzyme (ACE), and other products – plasminogen activator, prostacyclin, and thromboxane. Damaged endothelial cells cause apo-surfactant to be released to the systemic circulation.

Injury induces a proliferation of reactive cells. Macrophages, mononuclear cells, and more activated 'helper' T cells, possibly in response to TGF-β, contribute to a proliferation of fibroblasts. TGF-β is produced by both 'local' injured lung parenchyma as well as tumor site production of a de novo circulating serum component [Anscher et al., 1995]. TGF-β may directly influence gene expression of extracellular matrix molecules residing in stromal cells [Rodemann and Bamberg, 1995]. These stromal cells in turn contribute to the formation of collagen while inhibiting collagenase. Communication between fibroblasts and infiltrating T lymphocytes via the CD40 ligand pathway (a 50-kD member of the tumor necrosis factor-alpha receptor superfamily) promotes this activity also [Sempowski et al., 1997; Fries et al., 1995].

TGF-β may also accentuate fibroblast proliferation indirectly via stimulation of platelet-derived growth factor (PDGF). Moreover, TGF-β plays a critical role in autocrine stimulation of fibroblasts which can result in long-term activation and differentiation into a fibrotic phenotype via the premature terminal differentiation of this cell type [Rodemann and Bamberg, 1995]. The measurement of plasma TGF-β levels during treatment may help delineate the risk of developing radiation pneumonitis [Anscher et al., 1994, 1997].

Acute reactive cells are not found in either the interstitium or in the alveolar fluid. Macrophages normally function to clear debris from the alveolar space. Macrophages also seem to maintain surfactant homeostasis, and to take up surfactant released from type II cells and process it. After irradiation, type II cells degranulate and lose surfactant. The nadir level of macrophages are found about 21 days later [Travis and Komaki, 1996]. When the number of macrophages decreases, surfactant tends to accumulate in the alveolar space or be released to the systemic circulation through damaged endothelium. Macrophage number, control, and action are influenced by an array of factors. These cells play a role in protecting the lung from pneumonitis, and possibly as an accessory in the production of the thickening of septa in response to injury [Rodemann and Bamberg, 1995].

The association of an alveolar space that contains humidified air and is lined with type II cells, and the pulmonary capillary bed that is lined with the vascular endothelial cells, forms the acinus – the pulmonary functional subunit. It is clear we are endowed with redundant numbers of these functional units at birth, but the number is diminished and damaged over time. In chronic obstructive lung disease caused by tobacco use, there is decreased surface area for gas exchange, and the formation of bullae that have excess air and decreased surface area to exchange gases. Thus, functional subunits are lost. The terminal bronchiole functions by allowing the free diffusion of carbon dioxide into the alveolar space and the energy-dependent transport of oxygen from the air space back into the systemic circulation [Snell, 1996]. A decrease in the diffusion capacity is one indicator of damage to functional lung parenchyma [Abratt and Willcox, 1994].

The use of the metaphor of 'Christmas tree lights' helps to describe and understand the relations of functional subunits of normal tissues. There are two types of these electrical strings of Christmas lights. In one, the bulbs (which here represent the functional subunits) are arranged in series. When one bulb burns out, the entire strand goes dark. In the other, where the bulbs have a parallel circuit, when one bulb burns out, it is the only one that does. Those who have searched for the one burned out bulb in the in-series string remember this comparison well.

The lung, the liver and the kidney are examples of the 'in parallel' situation: a number of functional units can be lost before the loss becomes apparent [Marks, 1996]. For the Christmas tree, a few lights out on a multistrand set are undetectable to the casual eye. For the lung, loss of some terminal bronchioles will not be noticed until a critical number have been lost, after which the organ is impaired and the organism suffers. If loss continues beyond the critical level, death ensues. For normal tissues with an 'in series' arrangement, such as the gastrointestinal tract and the spinal cord, loss of one subunit causes complete dysfunction – intestinal perforation or loss of a central system nerve track – more problem than looking for the solitary burned out bulb on Christmas eve!

Clinical Treatment Issues Pertinent to Lung Cancer

Although most deaths from lung cancer are caused by systemic disease, local control remains an important issue. Most physicians believe that surgery is the best mode of obtaining local control, but too few patients can undergo surgery, and many that do still die of their lung cancer. Even those patients with small lesions, good performance status, few comorbid diseases and little weight loss can die from cancer after complete tumor resection. We are learning that there may be molecular markers that identify subsets of patients with poorer outcome [Minna, 1996].

Radiation oncology 'sits in the back seat' of lung cancer therapy because survival and local control have been poor with standard radiotherapy methods. Treatment has consisted of 60 Gy to a regional volume that included the primary tumor and the regional supraclavicular lymph nodes, mediastinal lymph nodes and an arbitrary 5 cm below the carina [Perez et al., 1982, 1987]. All too commonly contralateral hilar lymph nodes were included [Perez et al., 1982, 1987; Byhardt et al., 1993]. With this generous volume, often enlarged further to cover uncertainty of tumor extent, day-to-day variation in set-up, and physical and physiologic motion, the total dose has been limited by the radiation tolerance of the normal tissues. The usual practice has been to indicate this large volume to a dose of 40–50 Gy, then a smaller target volume to 60 Gy. With this approach the 5-year survival has averaged only 5%, and local control has been a paltry 8–20%. Because of these poor results, surgery has again been called upon for selected patients. Unfortunately, if there are pathologically proven lymph nodes in the mediastinum, survival is quite similar to radiotherapy, about 10% [Pearson, 1982].

Modern imaging has allowed for more precise and accurate identification of the primary tumor and regional lymph nodes. Despite this, radiotherapy practice has been slow to change; broad treatment of even radiographically negative areas continues to be a common practice. The frequency of cancer failure in involved areas versus failure in clinically uninvolved sites is not clear. One could argue that most local failure occurs in the area of initial bulk, and that increasing dose to the bulky tumor may bear more fruit than delivering largely ineffective doses to broader volumes that include nodes at risk but not clinically involved with cancer. Patients with nodes that are involved clinically or by surgical confirmation do have the largest risk of failing, but their failure pattern is at distant sites. Even when their local disease is controlled, subclinical distant metastases may already be present. Consequently, *we advocate maximizing radiotherapy to sites of known disease.*

Potential of Conformal Therapy

With the advent of computed tomography (CT), magnetic resonance imaging (MRI), and most recently, single photon emission computed tomography (SPECT), clinicians have been able to more precisely target visible tumor and better exclude normal dose-limiting tissues [Emami, 1996]. These imaging tools enable the clinician to visualize the target in multiple dimensions, permitting beam's eye view visualization, while CT and MRI help to delineate the visible tumor, SPECT lung perfusion assesses the physiological function at the vascular/alveolar interface [Marks et al., 1997; Boersma et al.,

1993]. This has facilitated attempts at dose escalation by allowing beam planning through areas of less functional lung. When the GTV (gross tumor volume, defined as radiographically visible tumor-appearing tissue) is treated to total doses of >70 Gy, toxicity does not necessarily worsen [Graham et al., 1995]. The St. Louis group has noted that there is no grade 3 or higher pneumonitis when 50% of the ipsilateral lung (the critical volume) receives <20 Gy (the threshold dose) [Graham et al., 1995]. Just as important however is the issue of locoregional control. Longer follow-up will determine if treating smaller and better defined tumor volumes to higher doses of radiation is superior to more conventional schemes, which have historically included clinically negative nodes within the treatment portals for prophylactic medication. Preliminary data would indicate that local in-field progression-free survival at least is not compromised by this change in philosophy [Hazuka et al., 1993].

The use of smaller fields also may allow more effective concomitant therapy with systemic agents. It has been frequently necessary to reduce chemotherapy doses when utilizing large radiation treatment portals because of excessive (often esophageal-related) toxicity. However, concomitant therapy appears to be superior to sequential treatment schemes for small cell lung cancer and potentially for locally advanced (stage II medically inoperable or stage III) non-small cell lung cancer [Turris, 1997; Komaki, 1996; Johnson et al., 1996]. A concern with the concomitant approach is the potential for increased pulmonary, esophageal and hematologic toxicity. These may be less likely to be life-threatening if cisplatin-based chemotherapy regimens are utilized instead of doxorubicin-based ones, and if traditional large radiotherapy portals are replaced by more deliberate targeting of the known disease.

In summary, we believe that the issue of what constitutes the necessary treatment target volume is paramount to the design of new clinical trials utilizing dose-escalation schemes of radiotherapy with or without concomitant chemotherapy. Of note, while classical radiation pneumonitis is likely to be decreased if smaller treatment volumes are used, the sporadic case of out-of-field radiation pneumonitis may not be effected to the same degree [Morgan et al., 1994].

As the complex mechanism of tissue fibrosis unfolds, it may well be possible to significantly reduce both acute and chronic sequelae of lung irradiation. Treating smaller volumes through less functional lung will potentially reduce the likelihood of injury to functional normal lung parenchyma. Novel selective inhibition of TGF-β production or CD40 may also decrease fibrogenesis and subsequent pulmonary fibrosis from radiation injury to normal lung parenchymal tissues [Fries et al., 1995; Border and Noble, 1994].

Acknowledgement

The authors express their thanks to Karen Capps for preparation of the manuscript.

References

Abratt RP, Willcox PA: Changes in lung function and perfusion after irradiation in patients with lung cancer. Lung Cancer 1994;11:61–69.

Anscher MS, Kong F-M, Marks LB, Bentel GC, Jirtle RL: Changes in plasma transforming growth factor beta during radiotherapy and the risk of symptomatic radiation-induced pneumonitis. Int J Radiat Oncol Biol Phys 1997;37:253–258.

Anscher MS, Kong F-M, Murase T, Jirtle RL: Short communication: Normal tissue injury after cancer therapy is a local response exacerbated by an endocrine effect of TGFβ. Br J Radiol 1995;68:331–333.

Anscher MS, Murase T, Prescott DM, Marks LB, Reisenbichler H, Bentel GC, Spencer D, Sherouse G, Jirtle RL: Changes in plasma TGFβ levels during pulmonary radiotherapy as a predictor of the risk of developing radiation pneumonitis. Int J Radiat Oncol Biol Phys 1994;30:671–676.

Arriagada R, Le Chevalier T, Rekacewicz C, Quoix E, De Cremoux H, Douillard JY, Tarayre M: Cisplatin-based chemotherapy in patients with locally advanced non-small cell lung cancer (NSCLC): Late analysis of a French randomized trial. Proc Am Soc Clin Oncol 1997;16:446.

Bleehen NM, Cox JD: Radiotherapy for lung cancer. Int J Radiat Oncol Biol Phys 1984;11:1001–1007.

Boersma LJ, Damen EMF, de Boer RW, Muller SH, Valdes Olmos RA, Hoefnagel CA, Roos CM, van Zandwijk N, Lebesque JV: A new method to determine dose-effect relations for local lung-function changes using correlated SPECT and CT data. Radiother Oncol 1993;29:110–116.

Border WA, Noble NA: Transforming growth factor β in tissue fibrosis. N Engl J Med 1994;331:1286–1292.

Byhardt RW, Martin L, Pajak TF, Shin KH, Emami B, Cox JD: The influence of field size and other treatment factors on pulmonary toxicity following hyperfractionated irradiation for inoperable non-small cell lung cancer (NSCLC) – Analysis of a Radiation Therapy Oncology Group (RTOG) protocol. Int J Radiat Oncol Biol Phys 1993;27:537–544.

Davis SD, Yankelevitz DF, Henschke CI: Radiation effects on the lung: Clinical features, pathology, and imaging findings. AJR 1992;159:1157–1164.

Emami B: Three-dimensional conformal radiation therapy in bronchogenic carcinoma. Semin Rad Oncol 1996;6:92–97.

Finkelstein JN, Johnston CJ, Baggs R, Rubin P: Early alterations in extracellular matrix and transforming growth factor beta gene expression in mouse lung indicative of late radiation fibrosis. Int J Radiat Oncol Biol Phys 1994;28:621–631.

Fries KM, Sempowski GD, Gaspari AA, Blieden T, Looney RJ, Phipps RP: CD-40 expression by human fibroblasts. Clin Immunol Immunopathol 1995;77:42–51.

Graham MV, Purdy JA, Emami B, Matthews JW, Harms WB: Preliminary results of a prospective trial using three-dimensional radiotherapy for lung cancer. Int J Radiat Oncol Biol Phys 1995;33:993–1000.

Hazuka MB, Turrisi AT III, Lutz ST, Martel MK, Ten Haken RK, Strawderman M, Borema PL, Lichter AS: Results of high-dose thoracic irradiation incorporating beam's eye view display in non-small cell lung cancer: A retrospective multivariate analysis. Int J Radiat Oncol Biol Phys 1993;27:273–284.

Johnson DH, Turrisi AT, Pass HI: Combined modality treatment for locally advanced non-small cell lung cancer; in Pass H, Mitchell JB, Johnson DH, Turrisi AT (eds): Lung Cancer: Principles and Practice. Philadelphia, Lippincott-Raven, 1996, pp 863–874.

Keng PC, Phipps R, Penney DP: In vitro radiation sensitivity of mouse lung fibroblasts isolated by flow cytometry. Int J Radiat Oncol Biol Phys 1995;31:519–523.

King RJ, Jones MB, Minoo P: Regulation of lung cell proliferation by polypeptide growth factors. Am J Physiol 1989;257:23.

Komaki R: Combined chemotherapy and radiation therapy in surgically unresectable regionally advanced non-small cell lung cancer. Semin Rad Oncol 1996;6:86–91.

Marks LB: The pulmonary effects of thoracic irradiation. Oncology 1994;8:89–100.

Marks LB: The impact of organ structure on radiation response. Int J Radiat Oncol Biol Phys 1996;34: 1165–1171.

Marks LB, Munley MT, Spencer DP, Sherouse GW, Bentel GC, Hoppenworth J, Chew M, Jaszczak RJ, Coleman RE, Prosnitz LR: Quantification of radiation-induced regional lung injury with perfusion imaging. Int J Radiat Oncol Biol Phys 1997;38:399–409.

Minna JD: Molecular biology: Overview; in Pass H, Mitchell JB, Johnson DH, Turrisi AT (eds): Lung Cancer: Principles and Practice. Philadelphia, Lippincott-Raven, 1996, pp 143–148.

Morgan GW, Pharm B, Breit SN: Radiation and the lung: A reevaluation of the mechanisms mediating pulmonary injury. Int J Radiat Oncol Biol Phys 1994;31:361–369.

Movsas B, Raffin TA, Epstein AH, Link CJ Jr: Pulmonary radiation injury. Chest 1997;111:1061–1076.

Pearson FG, Delarue NC, Ilves R, Todd TR, Cooper JD: Significance of positive superior mediastinal nodes identified at mediastinoscopy in patients with resectable cancer of the lung. J Thorac Cardiovasc Surg 1982;83:1–11.

Perez CA, Pajak TF, Rubin P, Simpson JR, Mohiuddin M, Brady LW, Perez-Tamayo R, Rotman M: Long-term observations of the patterns of failure in patients with unresectable nonoat cell carcinoma of the lung treated with definitive irradiation. Report by the Radiation Therapy Oncology Group. Cancer 1987;59:1874–1881.

Perez CA, Stanley K, Grundy G, Hanson W, Rubin P, Kramer S, Brady LW, Marks JE, Perez-Tamayo R, Brown GS, Concannon JP, Rotman M: Impact of irradiation technique and tumor extent in tumor control and survival of patients with unresectable nonoat cell carcinoma of the lung. Cancer 1982;50:1091–1099.

Phillips TL: An ultrastructural study of the development of radiation injury in the lung. Radiology 1966; 87:49–54.

Roach M III, Gandara DR, Yuo H-S, Swift PS, Kroll S, Shrieve DC, Wara WB, Margolis L, Phillips TL: Radiation pneumonitis following combined modality therapy for lung cancer: Analysis of prognostic factors. J Clin Oncol 1995;13:2606–2612.

Roberts CM, Foulcher E, Zaunders JJ, Bryant DH, Freund J, Cairns D, Penny R, Morgan GW, Breit SN: Radiation pneumonitis: A possible lymphocyte-mediated hypersensitivity reaction. Ann Intern Med 1993;118:696–700.

Rodemann HP, Bamberg M: Cellular basis of radiation-induced fibrosis. Radiother Oncol 1995;35:83–90.

Rubin P, Casarett GW: Clinical Radiation Pathology. Philadelphia, Saunders, 1968, vol 1, pp 423–470.

Rubin P, Finkelstein J, Shapiro D: Molecular biology mechanisms in the radiation induction of pulmonary injury syndromes: Interrelationship between the alveolar macrophage and the septal fibroblast. Int J Radiat Oncol Biol Phys 1992;24:93–101.

Rubin P, Johnston CJ, Williams JP, McDonald S, Finkelstein JN: A perpetual cascade of cytokines postirradiation leads to pulmonary fibrosis. Int J Radiat Oncol Biol Phys 1995;33:99–109.

Sempowski GD, Chess PR, Phipps RP: CD40 is a functional activation antigen and B7-independent T cell costimulatory molecule on normal human lung fibroblasts. J Immunol 1997;158:4670–4677.

Snell JD Jr: Normal lung physiology; in Pass H, Mitchell JB, Johnson DH, Turrisi AT (eds): Lung Cancer: Principles and Practice. Philadelphia, Lippincott-Raven, 1996, pp 409–420.

Travis EL, Komaki R: Treatment-related lung damage; in Pass H, Mitchell JB, Johnson DH, Turrisi AT (eds): Lung Cancer: Principles and Practice. Philadelphia, Lippincott-Raven, 1996, pp 285–301.

Turrisi AT III: Combined modality therapy for limited small cell lung cancer. Semin Rad Oncol 1997; 7(suppl 2):8–14.

Dr. Charles Thomas, Jr., Department of Radiation Oncology,
Medical University of South Carolina, Charleston, SC 29425 (USA)
Tel. +1 803 792 3273, Fax +1 803 792 5498, E-Mail thomas@radonc.musc.edu

Meyer JL (ed): Radiation Injury. Advances in Management and Prevention.
Front Radiat Ther Oncol. Basel, Karger, 1999, vol 32, pp 71–84

....

Radiation Injury to the Heart:
Risk Factors, Diagnosis,
Prevention and Treatment

J. Robert Stewart[a], *E. William Hancock*[b], *Steven L. Hancock*[c]

[a] Department of Radiation Oncology, University of Utah School of Medicine,
  Salt Lake City, Utah;
[b] Division of Cardiovascular Medicine and
[c] Department of Radiation Oncology, Stanford University, Stanford, Calif., USA

Introduction

The introduction and rapid adoption of high-energy therapeutic radiation sources in the 1950s and 1960s made dramatic changes in the role of radiation therapy for malignancies. The skin was no longer the organ limiting dose escalation, and a wide variety of deeply seated tumors could be irradiated to potentially cancericidal doses. Although supervoltage and megavoltage radiation beams facilitated effective treatment of tumors not often previously controlled by radiation, they also introduced new or previously unrecognized normal tissue complications. Cardiac damage, particularly pericardial damage, became appreciated when high-energy radiation fields were applied to tumors adjacent to the heart or to thoracic volumes at risk for tumor that included the heart [1]. Table 1 summarizes the various classes of cardiac complications seen after radiotherapy. In general, acute abnormalities, such as acute pericarditis arising during the course of radiation or various physiological changes observed during radiation, are transient, do not presage clinically important late damage, and will not be discussed further here. The early descriptions of cardiac disease after irradiation focused on pericardial disease, which may present either as acute pericarditis or as a pericardial effusion with or without tamponade. A small fraction of patients developed pericardial constriction. Myocardial injury was usually associated with clinically dominant pericardial disease and became recognized when patients with apparent constrictive or restrictive pericardial disease did not improve after undergoing pericardiec-

Table 1. Spectrum of delayed RIHD syndromes

Pericardial disease	Acute pericarditis with or without tamponade
	Pericardial effusion with or without tamponade
	Pericardial constriction
Myocardial disease	Pancarditis (high-dose radiation alone)
	Cardiomyopathy (chemotherapy – radiation)
Pleuro-pulmonary-cardiopathy	
Coronary artery disease	
Other	Valve defects, conduction abnormality

tomy and often had 'pancarditis' with signs of diffuse endocardial, myocardial, and pericardial fibrosis at autopsy. Cardiomyopathy, or an isolated myocardial injury, has been more commonly observed with anthracycline chemotherapeutic agents than with irradiation alone. However, clinical and animal data suggest that radiation and anthracyclines have additive adverse effects on the myocardium.

Early descriptions of precocious coronary artery disease in irradiated patients raised the question of a causal effect [1, 2]. More recent studies comparing the risk of coronary artery disease mortality in populations of treated populations with mortality in general populations show convincingly that it is an important potential risk after radiotherapy.

A variety of other cardiac problems have been observed in patients after cardiac irradiation. Valvular heart disease is probably more prevalent in irradiated patients, although the extent of this risk has not been firmly established. Conduction system abnormalities have clearly been observed and are likely related to myocardial fibrosis and distortion or interruption of the conduction bundles. The chronic pleural effusions that arise in some patients as late complications of mediastinal irradiation present a particularly vexing clinical problem. The etiology of such problems is often multifactorial and may derive from constrictive or restrictive pericardial disease, diminished cardiac muscle function, primary pleural disorders or putative lymphatic insufficiency in the irradiated mediastinum.

The observation and study of patients with late cardiac injuries after irradiation have led to a number of changes in technique designed to minimize such risks for future generations of patients. The purpose of this paper is to discuss the risk factors, diagnosis, prevention, and treatment of cardiac complications with an emphasis on technical approaches to facilitate prevention.

Table 2. Dose-response pericarditis in patients treated definitively at Stanford University, University of California at San Francisco, at risk at least 1 year, based on data reported by Stewart and Fajardo [9]

Dose, cGy	Stanford (n=318)		Combined Stanford-UCSF (n=411)	
	n	% pericarditis	n	% pericarditis
<3,500	0	0	37	0
3,500–4,000	6	0	43	2.2
4,000–4,500	270	7	280	6
4,500–5,000	30	10	33	7
>5,000	12	33	12	25

Pericardial and Myocardial Injury

An extensive literature describes various aspects of the pericardial and myocardial complications that may follow radiation therapy [1–8]. Clinical studies and prospective animal studies have given considerable insight into the relative contributions of dose and volume of irradiation to the risk of subsequent injury. Table 2 demonstrates the relationship between radiation dose and the subsequent incidence of clinical pericarditis observed in patients with Hodgkin's disease treated at Stanford University and University of California at San Francisco [9]. A clear dose response was seen with no cases observed at doses <3,500 cGy. Most of the patients in the series were treated to cardiac doses of 4,000–4,500 cGy with an incidence of 6%; doses >5,000 cGy increased the incidence to 25%. This dose response has been confirmed by other clinical studies and by studies of radiation-induced pericarditis in New Zealand white rabbits.

Many of the papers describing pericardial disease after irradiation focused on patients who had been treated for Hodgkin's disease. Extended field treatment of Hodgkin's disease frequently entailed radiation to significant volumes of the heart, and most of the patients were cured or achieved prolonged survivals that allowed cardiac complications to become manifest. Early treatment approaches to Hodgkin's disease frequently featured techniques in which all or most of the heart was included in the portals for all of the course of treatment. In some institutions, opposed anterior and posterior mediastinal treatment fields were weighted from the anterior field or an unopposed anterior field was used with doses calculated to the middle of the mediastinum. It was common practice to treat only one field per day in opposed anterior and posterior portal treatments. These approaches gave the heart a high dose per fraction and gave high total doses to the anterior pericardium and the right

Table 3. Effect of blocking cardiac apex and the subcarinal heart block [12]

Cardiac shielding	Incidence of pericarditis
None	20%
Left ventricular block	7%
Subcarinal block after 30 Gy	2.5%

ventricular and anterior left ventricular walls. The total doses used frequently exceeded what is now considered cardiac tolerance. From these early studies it is apparent that the dose per fraction is important. Patients treated with anterior only or anteriorly weighted fields had a higher incidence of pericarditis than those treated with techniques that achieved more homogeneous dose distributions [8, 11]. Early reports of cardiac injury also demonstrated a correlation between total radiation dose to the heart and the severity of injury. For example, of the 10 Stanford patients with pancarditis reported in 1971, 8 had received doses ranging from 6,000 to 9,800 cGy [9]. The effect of cardiac volume irradiated upon subsequent risk of pericarditis was also demonstrated in a report from Stanford comparing patients irradiated for Hodgkin's disease, who had most or all of their heart in the field, with patients treated for breast cancer, who, at that time, were treated with techniques that included 20–30% of the heart in the field [9]. The doses associated with a 5% incidence of pericarditis were in the range of 4,000 cGy for large heart volumes and 6,000 cGy for smaller volumes. Table 3, based on data reported by Carmel and Kaplan [12] in 1976, speaks directly to the effect of volume on the risk of pericardial injury. Excluding part of the left ventricle from the mediastinal radiation field used in Hodgkin's disease decreased the incidence from 20 to 7%, and blocking of the subcarinal area after 30 Gy decreased the incidence further to 2.5%. A subsequent study comparing the risk for heart disease death among patients treated for Hodgkin's disease at Stanford with general population risks [13] showed that these changes in blocking techniques decreased the relative risk of death from 5.5 to 1.7 (not significantly elevated) for cardiac deaths other than myocardial infarction.

The treatment of Hodgkin's disease has evolved so that radiation doses now seldom exceed the pericardial injury threshold dose of approximately 4,000 cGy. Radiation fields are shaped to exclude at least a part of the heart volume for at least part of the treatment. There is also more frequent use of partial transmission blocking which reduces both the dose to the part of the heart underlying such blocks and the dose per fraction. In patients with large mediastinal masses, initial chemotherapy often reduces the size of the mass, allowing smaller radiation portal volumes and often smaller cardiac volumes.

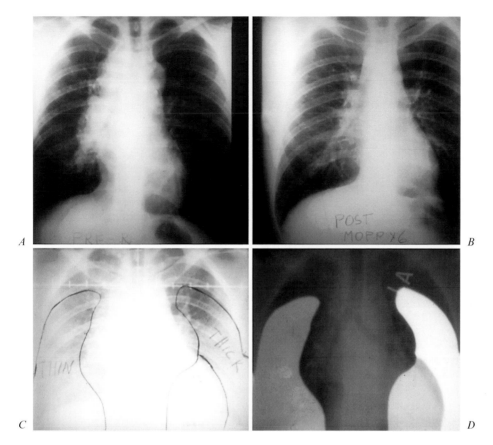

A

B

C

D

Fig. 1. Twenty-year-old man with stage IIB Hodgkin's disease involving bilateral supra-clavicular, mediastinal and right hilar adenopathy. *A* Pretreatment X-ray. *B* Chest X-ray following 6 cycles of MOPP chemotherapy. *C* Simulation planning film specifying 50% transmission block to the right lung and cardiac apex with full-thickness block to the remaining left lung. *D* Treatment portal showing these blocks.

Elements of the approach to Hodgkin's disease at the University of Utah in recent decades are shown in figures 1–4. With consistent application of these approaches, the complications of pericarditis and pancarditis has essentially disappeared from practice.

Pericardial Disease, Clinical Aspects and Treatment

Pericardial disease caused by radiation is similar to typical idiopathic or viral pericarditis and to the pericarditis observed after pericardiotomy. Acute pericarditis is manifested chiefly as pleuritic midline anterior chest pain, a

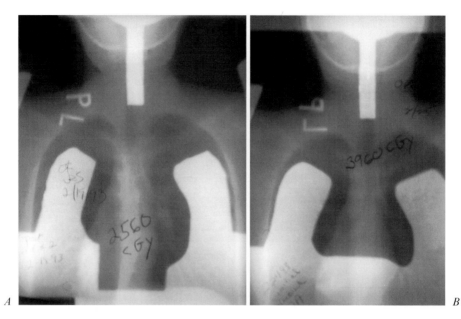

A   B

Fig. 2. Seventeen-year-old woman with stage IIA Hodgkin's disease involving the supra-clavicular nodes bilaterally, and the upper right mediastinum. *A* A posterior portal showing the blocking for the first 2,560 cGy with the cardiac apex excluded. *B* The remade lung blocks including the blocking of the subcarinal area. This portal was then carried to a total dose of 3,960 cGy.

pericardial friction rub, and a pattern of diffuse ST segment elevation in the electrocardiogram. Pericardial effusion may or may not be present. Acute pericarditis is usually benign and self-limited. Treatment is symptomatic, and usually consists of aspirin or nonsteroidal anti-inflammatory agents. Cortico-steroids are more dramatically effective as symptomatic therapy, but should be reserved for the small number of severe and persistent cases because of the risk of steroid dependency and relapses of acute pericarditis when they are withdrawn.

Chronic pericardial effusion is usually asymptomatic, and is discovered in a routine follow-up chest radiograph. Tamponade is not usually present, because the pericardium stretches when an effusion develops slowly. These patients can usually be managed by observation alone, with the expectation that the effusion will resolve, or will persist in a benign form.

Cardiac tamponade occurs in some cases of acute pericarditis with effusion or chronic pericardial effusion. It should be suspected when dyspnea is present, and can be confirmed by demonstrating elevated jugular venous pressure,

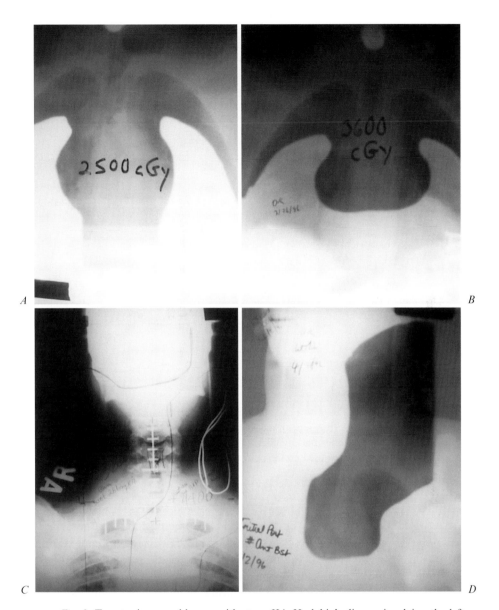

Fig. 3. Twenty-six-year-old man with stage IIA Hodgkin's disease involving the left neck, supraclavicular and left upper mediastinal nodes. *A* the initial blocking of the mantle field which was carried to 2,500 cGy. *B* The remade blocks to exclude the subcarinal area. This was carried to 3,600 cGy. *C* The simulator film for the final boost field to the upper mediastinum and left neck. *D* The treatment portal. This area of bulk disease was carried to 4,400 cGy.

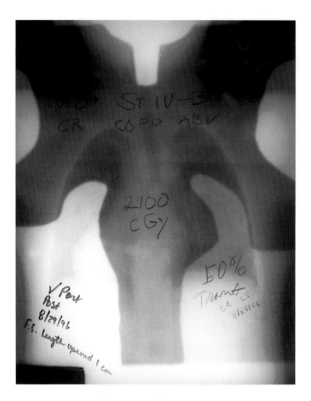

Fig. 4. Posterior portal of a typical set-up in a pediatric patient. This 9-year-old boy had stage IVB Hodgkin's disease with mediastinal, neck, and right lung involvement. The photo is a copy of a posterior port film illustrating the volume carried to 2,100 cGy. A 50% transmission lung block was used on the right side. Cardiac apex was excluded throughout.

usually with a paradoxical pulse if carefully looked for. Echocardiography is necessary to demonstrate the effusion, and is also helpful, but not necessarily definitive, in assessing the presence of tamponade. Cardiac tamponade should be managed by removal of the fluid. Usually, a needle pericardiocentesis is the preferred initial approach. Pericardiostomy or partial pericardiectomy by a subxiphoid, thoracoscopic, or thoracotomy approach are more definitive procedures, which may be selected for initial management in some cases. Complicated cases in which pericardial effusion and constrictive pericarditis are both present (effusive-constrictive pericarditis) require hemodynamic assessment by cardiac catheterization combined with pericardiocentesis.

Constrictive pericarditis usually presents as a syndrome of right-sided fluid retention with diminished effort tolerance. Recognition of elevated jugular venous pressure, combined with demonstration of normal size and wall motion of both ventricles, is the key to recognizing constriction. Cardiac catheterization, to demonstrate elevated and equilibrated diastolic pressures in the two ventricles, and CT or MRI of the thorax to demonstrate thickened pericardium, usually provide sufficient confirmation. Pericardiectomy is the only definitive therapy, but is a procedure with significant operative mortality risk. Patients with past radiotherapy should be selected for pericardiectomy particularly carefully, because the often associated myocardial, pulmonary, and pleural pathology increase the risk and limit the value of the operation in many instances. Patients with these associated problems in whom the fluid retention may be well controlled by diuretic therapy are sometimes better managed without attempting pericardiectomy. With current techniques of radiotherapy we would expect less myocardial damage; if constriction does occur in patients treated with the new techniques, surgical results may well be better.

Radiation pericardial and myocardial injury can occur in patients with breast cancer, lung cancer, or esophageal cancer. In breast cancer one should avoid direct photon irradiation of the internal mammary nodes [14]. If the target volume overlies the heart, electrons should be used to spare dose to the heart. Tangential portals used to treat left-sided breast cancers should be carefully designed to exclude the heart. In other cancers in the chest it is often possible to reduce cardiac dose by delivering part of the tumor dose by lateral or oblique ports that miss the cardiac ventricles.

Coronary Artery Disease

The first report from Stanford concerning radiation-induced heart disease [1] included one case of a 14-year-old boy with a fatal myocardial infarction. Over the ensuing years, a number of other cases were described that raised the question of an association between mediastinal irradiation and subsequent coronary artery disease [2, 15]. More recently, the Stockholm trial comparing postoperative radiation therapy with surgery alone for breast cancer showed an excess mortality due to coronary artery disease in the women receiving high-dose radiation to the heart as part of postoperative treatment of carcinoma of the breast [16]. Excess coronary artery disease mortality was also noted in a follow-up study of patients treated for Hodgkin's disease [17]. In 1993, papers reviewing cases of coronary artery disease in children and adults [13, 18] treated at Stanford for Hodgkin's disease convincingly showed an excess mortality from coronary artery disease. At this time there can be little doubt that cardiac irradiation is a risk factor for subsequent development of coronary artery disease.

Table 4. Risks for death from acute myocardial infarction following treatment of Hodgkin's disease (2,232 patients; 21,164 person-years of observation)

Group	Observed/ expected events	Relative risk	95% confidence intervals	Absolute risk
All patients	55/17.3	3.2	2.3–4.0	17.8
Males	47/14.3	3.3	2.3–4.2	27.0
Females	8/3.0	2.6	1.2–5.0	5.5

Table 5. Risks for death from acute myocardial infarction according to treatment of Hodgkin's disease

Group	Observed/ expected events	Relative risk	95% confidence intervals	Absolute risk
Radiation alone (including mediastinum)	35/8.4	4.1	2.8–5.5	25.7
Combined treatment (mediastinum irradiated)	14/5.2	2.7	1.5–3.8	9.7
No mediastinal irradiation (CT/RT alone or combined)	6/3.6	1.7	0.7–3.5	–

In their 1993 paper, Hancock et al. [13] assessed the risk of heart disease following radiation therapy for Hodgkin's disease in a retrospective analysis of the 2,232 consecutive patients treated at Stanford between 1960 and 1991. The average follow-up was 9.5 years. The relative risk of death from coronary artery disease was assessed by comparing the treated study patients with matched general population controls. Some of the data from that study are shown in tables 4–8. There were 55 deaths due to acute myocardial infarction which gave a relative risk of 3.2 for the entire population. The risk was somewhat higher in males than in females (table 4). Combining chemotherapy with radiotherapy did not increase the relative risk of coronary artery disease (table 5). Cardiac doses $\leqslant 30$ Gy were not associated with a statistically significant increased relative risk, and reducing volume for part of the treatment (as was seen in patients treated after 1972) did not significantly decrease the relative risk of coronary artery mortality (table 6). Even with extensive cardiac blocking at least the proximal coronary arteries are in the field when the mediastinum is treated (fig. 1). Age at the time of radiation is an important determinant of risk for coronary artery disease, with the relative risk for patients treated between the ages of 10 and 19 being 44.7. By age 50 or greater the increased relative risk largely disappeared (table 7). Relative risk also

Table 6. Risks for death from acute myocardial infarction according to extent of mediastinal irradiation for Hodgkin's disease

Group	Observed/expected events	Relative risk	95% confidence intervals	Absolute risk
Mediastinal dose >0 and ≤30 Gy	2/0.5	4.2	0.7–13.8	–
Mediastinal dose >30 Gy	47/13.3	3.5	2.5–4.5	18.6
Mediastinal irradiation before 1972	26/7.0	3.7	2.3–5.1	24.7
Mediastinal irradiation after 1972	23/6.8	3.4	2.0–4.8	13.9

Table 7. Effect of age at irradiation on risks of acute myocardial infarction (AMI) death following treatment of Hodgkin's disease

Age at irradiation years	Observed/expected events	Relative risk (RR)[1]	95% confidence intervals	Absolute risk (AR)*,[1]
<10	0/0.002	–	–	–
10–19	6/0.13	44.7	18.0–93.0	12.4
20–29	8/1.1	7.3	3.4–13.8	9.0
30–39	14/2.7	5.1	2.9–7.4	27.4
40–49	9/3.0	3.0	1.4–5.5	43.6
≥50	12/6.8	1.8	1.0–3.0	–

* Absolute risk is expressed as excess cases per 10,000 person-years.
[1] χ for trend in AMI-RR: $p \leq 0.0001$; χ for trend in AMI-AR: 2.6, $p = 0.01$.

increased with increasing time following irradiation (table 8). Similar conclusions were reached in a smaller study by King et al. [19].

What steps can be taken to respond to these risk factors with an aim toward prevention? In adolescents and young adults with Hodgkin's disease, reducing the total dose seems warranted. In that population a higher reliance on chemotherapy combined with lower dose irradiation has been adopted by many centers and should decrease cardiovascular mortality. Although partial shielding of the heart has not significantly reduced the relative risk of acute myocardial infarction death after mediastinal irradiation, the blocking techniques used probably offered little protection of the proximal coronary arteries. There may be a role for more sophisticated treatment planning to reduce the radiation dose to the aortic root and proximal coronary arteries in some patients. Coronary artery disease is a multifactorial process with genetic,

Table 8. Latency of risk for acute myocardial infarction (AMI) death after treatment of Hodgkin's disease

Years after initial Hodgkin's disease Tx	Observed/expected events	Relative risk[1]	95% confidence intervals	Absolute risk*,[1]
0–4	12/6.0	2.0	1.1–3.3	6.4
5–9	17/4.7	3.6	2.2–4.5	20.1
10–14	11/3.7	3.0	1.6–5.2	20.5
15–19	11/2.2	5.0	2.6–8.7	54.2
≥20	4/0.7	5.6	1.8–13.6	70.6

* Absolute risk is expressed as excess cases per 10,000 person-years.
[1] χ for trend in relative risk of AMI death: 2.3, p=0.02; χ for trend in absolute risk of AMI death: 3.8, p=0.0002.

dietary and lifestyle risk factors. Certainly, patients who have had significant cardiac irradiation exposure should be counselled to minimize other potential cardiac risk factors, such as smoking, lipid and cholesterol abnormalities.

Another strategy for decreasing mortality might be screening for occult disease and treating before there is serious morbidity. Currently at Stanford a study is underway to evaluate the effect of screening of previously treated Hodgkin's patients. Screening begins with a careful history for suspicious symptoms. Patients accepted to the study are then screened with a fasting lipid profile and exercise stress tests using echocardiography and sestimibi or thallium scans with angiography for confirmation of suspected coronary artery disease. So far, 202 patients have been screened, 11% of whom had positive stress tests. Among 19 patients who have completed subsequent angiography, 7 had severe coronary artery disease. Four underwent coronary artery bypass grafts at age 29–52, 2 had angioplasties, and 1 refused bypass grafting. There may well be a role for other approaches to improve coronary artery blood flow such as coronary stenting [20], especially for proximal coronary stenosis.

Other Cardiac Effects

Valve Defects

Disease involving any of the four cardiac valves has been reported in the long-term follow-up after radiotherapy. The causative relation is less well substantiated than in the case of pericardial and coronary artery disease. The valvular pathology is similar to that of late inactive rheumatic heart disease, and consists of fibrous scarring of the leaflets that causes varying mixtures of stenosis and regurgitation. The disease is often mild, but a few patients have come to valve replacement surgery. As in rheumatic heart disease, the aortic and mitral valves are far more often affected than the tricuspid or pulmonary valves.

Conducting Abnormality

Atrioventricular conduction block has occurred in a small number of patients with past radiotherapy. The block is usually situated in the ventricles, involving the Purkinje branches. In such cases, bundle branch block usually develops first, providing a means of early detection and anticipation of later AV block in routine electrocardiograms. In other instances the AV block is situated in the AV node, and is preceded by prolongation of the PR interval. Implantation of a permanent pacemaker is indicated if the AV block causes symptoms, or if it is located in the His-Purkinje system (suggested by prior bundle branch block, the presence of Mobitz Type 2 incomplete AV block, or a notably slow idioventricular escape rhythm in complete AV block). Periodic electrocardiograms are indicated in the long-term follow-up of radiotherapy patients, particularly those with evidence of other forms of cardiac damage.

Miscellaneous

Patients with past radiotherapy sometimes demonstrate a chronic sinus tachycardia, with a resting heart rate of 90–100/min. The phenomenon is similar to that seen in patients with heart transplants, and probably reflects a degree of denervation of the heart. This condition appears to be benign, and need not be taken to indicate decompensation of other cardiac conditions that may be present.

Patients with past radiotherapy sometimes demonstrate chronic pleural effusions that appear to be out of proportion to the associated cardiac or pulmonary disease, if any. This calls for a more thorough than usual assessment for occult heart disease. However, it appears that a predilection for primary idiopathic pleural effusion may be present, perhaps caused by loss of some of the mediastinal lymphatic vessels that normally drain the pleural cavities.

References

1   Cohn KE, Stewart JR, Fajardo LF, Hancock W: Heart disease following radiation. Medicine 1967; 46:281–298.
2   Fajardo LF: Radiation-induced coronary artery disease (editorial). Chest 1977;71:563–564.
3   Stewart JR, Fajardo LF, Gillette SM, Constine LS: Radiation injury to the heart. Int J Radiat Oncol Biol Phys 1995;31:1205–1211.
4   Fajardo LF, Stewart JR, Cohn KE: Morphology of radiation-induced heart disease. Arch Pathol 1968;86:512–519.

5   Fajardo LF, Stewart JR: Pathogenesis of radiation-induced myocardial fibrosis. Lab Invest 1973; 29:244–257.

6   Gottdeiner JS, Katin MJ, Borer JS, Bachrach SL, Green MV: Late cardiac effects of therapeutic mediastinal irradiation: Assessment by echocardiography and radionuclide angiography. N Engl J Med 1983;308:569–572.

7   Brosius FC, Waller BF, Roberts WG: Radiation heart disease: Analysis of 16 young (aged 15–33 years) necropsy patients who received over 3,500 rads to the heart. Am J Med 1981;70:519–530.

8   Byhardt R, Brace K, Rukdeschel J, Chang P, Martin R, Wiernik P: Dose and treatment factors in radiation-related pericardial effusion associated with the mantle technique for Hodgkin's disease. Cancer 1975;35:795–802.

9   Stewart JR, Fajardo LF: Dose response in human and experimental radiation-induced heart disease. Application of the nominal standard dose concept. Radiology 1971;99:403–408.

10 Stewart JR: Normal tissue tolerance to irradiation of the cardiovascular system. Front Radiat Ther Oncol 1989;23:302–309.

11 Morton DL, Glancy DL, Joseph WL, Adkins PC: Management of patients with radiation-induced pericarditis with effusion: A note on the development of aortic regurgitation in two of them. Chest 1973;64:291–297.

12 Carmel RJ, Kaplan HS: Mantle irradiation in Hodgkin's disease. Cancer 1976;37:2813–2815.

13 Hancock SL, Tucker MA, Hoppe RT: Factors affecting late mortality from heart disease after treatment of Hodgkin's disease. JAMA 1993;270:1949–1955.

14 Harris JR, Hellman S: Put the 'hockey stick' on ice. Int J Radiat Oncol Biol Phys 1988;15:497–499.

15 Kopelson G, Herwig KJ: The etiologies of coronary artery disease in cancer patients. Int J Radiat Oncol Biol Phys 1978;4:895–906.

16 Rutqvist LE, Lax I, Fornander T, Johansson H: Cardiovascular mortality in a randomized trial of adjuvant radiation therapy vs surgery alone in primary breast cancer. Int J Radiat Oncol Biol Phys 1992;22:887–896.

17 Boivin JF, Hutchison GB, Lubin JH, Mauch P: Coronary artery disease mortality in patients treated for Hodgkin's disease. Cancer 1992;69:1241–1247.

18 Hancock SL, Donaldson SS: Radiation-related cardiac disease: Risks after treatment of Hodgkin's disease during childhood and adolescence; in Proceedings of Second International Conference on the Long-Term Complications of Treatment of Children and Adolescents for Cancer, Buffalo, NY, June 12–14, 1992.

19 King V, Constine LS, Clark D, Schwartz RG, Muhs AG, Henzler M, Hutson A, Rubin P: Symptomatic coronary artery disease after mantle irradiation for Hodgkin's disease. Int J Radiat Oncol Biol Phys 1996;36:881–889.

20 Versaci F, Gaspardone A, Tomai F, Crea F, Chiariello L, Gioffre PA: A comparison of coronary-artery stenting with angioplasty for isolated stenosis of the proximal left anterior descending coronary artery. N Engl J Med 1997;336:817–822.

J. Robert Stewart, MD, Department of Radiation Oncology, University of Utah, Health Science Center, 50 N Medical Drive, Salt Lake City, UT 84132 (USA)

Meyer JL (ed): Radiation Injury. Advances in Management and Prevention.
Front Radiat Ther Oncol. Basel, Karger, 1999, vol 32, pp 85–97

....

Prevention of Diagnostic and Treatment-Related Sequelae in Stage I and II Hodgkin's Disease

James D. Cox, Chul S. Ha

Department of Radiation Oncology, The University of Texas M.D. Anderson
Cancer Center, Houston, Tex., USA

Introduction

Hodgkin's disease (HD) is one of the great success stories of modern
oncology. In the 10th edition (1959) of Cecil and Loebs' Textbook of Medicine
[1], the hematologist Carl Moore stated: 'The disease is regarded as being
uniformly fatal, although a few isolated instances of apparent cure from early
excision and treatment of a primary site have been reported.' Thus portrayed
as categorically incurable, HD is now recognized as one of the most curable
forms of cancer. The reasons for this dramatically altered view are simple:
both radiation therapy for early disease and combination chemotherapy for
advanced disease are able to eliminate all evidence of HD in the majority of
cases. This has resulted not only in consistent increases in 5-year survival rates
in referral institutions (fig. 1), but also a highly significant decrease in annual
mortality rates in the USA since the early 1970s [2].

Recognition of the principles behind effective radiation therapy of HD
evolved slowly. The pioneering work of Rene Gilbert of Geneva, Switzerland,
and Vera Peters of Toronto, Canada, went unrecognized or was disbelieved.
Gilbert [3] made two pivotal observations: (1) if irradiation to affected lymph
nodes was stopped when the mass disappeared, the tumor often recurred, and
(2) if irradiation was confined only to involved lymph nodes, disease reappeared
in adjacent nodal sites. By continuing irradiation to higher total doses than
those required to cause a 'complete response', he found it possible to prevent
recurrence. By irradiating uninvolved nodal regions prophylactically, he
showed that adjacent relapses could be eliminated and long-term freedom

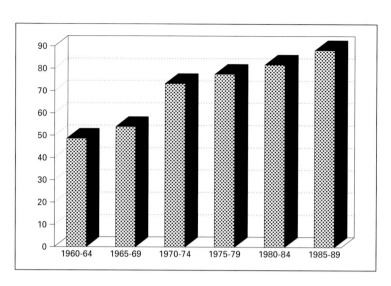

Fig. 1. Five-year survival rates for previously untreated patients with HD, all stages, treated at The University of Texas M.D. Anderson Cancer Center.

from relapse (FFR) could be achieved. Peters [4] treated a large series of patients with these principles and reported results as a function of initial extent of disease (stage) with impressive long-term survival even by today's standards. Henry Kaplan and Saul Rosenberg of Stanford University elaborated upon these concepts and promoted them among the radiation oncology and hematology/oncology communities in the 1960s. A key element of the educational process was a cooperative clinical trial in which major institutions in the USA and Canada participated [5]. The efforts of Rosenberg and Kaplan [6] gradually led to widespread adoption of more extensive and intensive irradiation for early HD than previously had been the practice in the USA.

Effective combination chemotherapy developed as investigators found it possible to combine agents shown to be effective singly, into regimens with doses and schedules that minimized toxicity to any given organ. Mustargen, vincristine, procarbazine and prednisone (MOPP), developed by DeVita and coworkers at the National Cancer Institute [7], proved to be strikingly effective and indeed curative of patients with advanced HD [8]. Within a decade, durable remissions were reported with a combination of doxorubicin, bleomycin, vinblastine and dacarbazine (ABVD) in patients who had proven resistant to MOPP [9]. In the ensuing years, the vast majority of patients have been treated with MOPP, ABVD, or combinations and modifications of these regimens.

The Stanford investigators also promoted the use of exploratory laparotomy [10] in addition to bipedal lymphography. They reasoned that the difference between disease confined to one side of the diaphragm (Ann Arbor [11] stages I and II) versus disease on both sides of the diaphragm (Ann Arbor stage III) was so important that this major surgical procedure was necessary to identify occult disease in the suprarenal para-aortic lymph nodes and spleen in addition to confirming lymphographic findings. Reported results have shown that approximately 30% of patients with stage I and II supradiaphragmatic presentations have evidence of HD below the diaphragm disclosed by laparotomy [12] which has justified the use of combination chemotherapy for many oncologists.

As successful evaluation and treatment has led to a growing number of patients free of HD and presumably cured, it became increasingly apparent that late consequences of some of these medical interventions were not rare and could be life-threatening or lethal. It therefore seems appropriate and timely to explore the most serious of the consequences of medical interventions for HD with a view toward minimizing adverse consequences. In the following discussion, a position will be taken that continued successful management of HD can be accomplished with decreased risks of adverse outcomes from management. These include: (1) omitting laparotomy as a routine staging procedure; (2) omitting chemotherapy for favorable patients with HD; (3) limiting doses with irradiation, and (4) limiting irradiation in patients treated with chemotherapy.

By following these policies, only procedures demonstrated to improve outcome will be used and the risks of leukemia and second malignant tumors will be kept to a minimum.

Laparotomy

Although initial presentations of early HD below the diaphragm are infrequent ($<5\%$), involvement of para-aortic lymph nodes and spleen is common. Infradiaphragmatic involvement can be assessed by bipedal lymphography (LAG), computed tomography (CT) or laparotomy (LAP). LAG has advantages over CT in that abnormal internal architecture can be demonstrated in lymph nodes of normal size [13]; CT has advantages over LAG in that the spleen and suprarenal para-aortic lymph nodes can be imaged. Marglin and Castellino [14] found a high degree of correlation between lymphography and laparotomy. CT and lymphography can be considered complementary: both are minimally invasive and carry no risk except allergic reactions to the contrast agent.

LAP has revealed infradiaphragmatic involvement in approximately 30% of patients with clinical stage I and II HD. A compilation of laparotomy data

[12] from five large series with a total of 2,431 clinical stage I and II patients showed that 72% of patients could be classified as stage I and II after LAP: approximately 26% were stage III and 2% were stage IV. On the surface, this seems justification alone for continuing staging LAP, but there are serious consequences of the procedure beside the costs, and there is not one shred of evidence that it improves survival or freedom from relapse.

The morbidity of LAP has been summarized thoroughly by Mendenhall [15]. She noted the finite risk of death or serious morbidity from anesthesia, subsequent bowel obstruction, overwhelming postsplenectomy infection (now largely preventable with vaccination), and the possible contribution of splenic absence to the risk of leukemia in these patients. If these risks were balanced by improvements in survival, the procedure might continue to be justified, but, no such evidence exists.

The European Organization for Research in the Treatment of Cancer (EORTC) has conducted a remarkable series of prospective trials in HD. The H2 trial [16], conducted between 1972 and 1976, compared the effectiveness of splenic irradiation with that of splenectomy in patients with clinical stages I and II. All patients received supradiaphragmatic irradiation using the mantle technique and all had para-aortic irradiation. Half the patients underwent laparotomy and splenectomy and half received splenic irradiation at the time of para-aortic treatment. Chemotherapy was administered to patients with HD with mixed cellularity or lymphocyte depletion. A total of 300 patients were enrolled in this trial. The actuarial survival and relapse-free survival rates were virtually identical. A successor trial (H6F) [17] refined the question to ask if the systematic use of combination chemotherapy in addition to irradiation in patients with positive LAP improved outcome over mantle, para-aortic and splenic irradiation (subtotal nodal irradiation, STNI) in clinically staged patients with favorable prognostic factors. With 262 patients enrolled in the two arms of the study, there again proved to be no significant differences in survival or relapse-free survival (fig. 2). In addition, 3 patients died of complications related to treatment in the LAP arm whereas there were no treatment-related deaths in the clinically staged patients.

Thus, the systematic use of chemotherapy in patients with advanced to pathologic stage III has not improved survival. Lesser justifications than improved outcome could be invoked to continue to advocate LAP. To date, however, they have not been sustained. LAP does not assure that transdiaphragmatic failures can be avoided when only mantle irradiation is used [18]. Omitting LAP is not associated with an increased risk of pelvic failures following STNI [19].

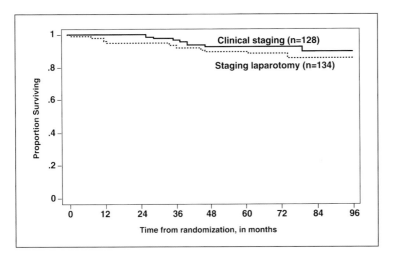

Fig. 2. EORTC H6F trial: Overall survival by treatment group. log rank test: p=0.24. (Reprinted with permission from Carde et al. [17].)

Chemotherapy

STNI is highly effective in favorable patients with stage I and II HD. Investigators in the EORTC Lymphoma Cooperative Group have identified favorable prognostic factors to be absence of systemic ('B') symptoms or an elevated erythrocyte sedimentation rate (ESR), age <50 years, involvement of <4 lymph node regions, and mediastinal mass/thoracic ratio <0.35 [20]. The addition of chemotherapy to STNI in these patients does not improve outcome.

Combination chemotherapy carries risks which are certainly warranted in less favorable patients. The risks of life-threatening granulocytopenia during treatment are low, but risks of late effects are considerable [21]. Myelodysplastic syndromes and acute leukemia, second malignant tumors, sterility, and long-term pulmonary and cardiac compromise have been well described. Much of the available literature concerning late effects is based on combination chemotherapy with mechlorethamine, vincristine (Oncovin), prednisone and procarbazine (MOPP). The use of a combination of doxorubicin (Adriamycin), bleomycin, vinblastine and dacarbazine (ABVD) is considered to have lessened the risks of leukemia and gonadal dysfunction, but has not eliminated them. The relative contributions of chemotherapy and radiation therapy to second malignant tumors will be considered further below.

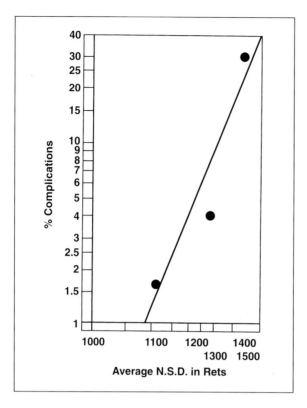

Fig. 3. Percent symptomatic pneumonitis, pericarditis, and myelitis as a function of dose. Dose expressed in rets (40 Gy in 20 fractions in 29 days = 1,340 rets). (Reprinted with permission from Fazekas et al. [22].)

Radiation Therapy

The entire body of data presented at this conference and included within the chapters of this publication attest to the potentially serious consequences of radiation therapy on normal tissues. This is especially relevant for young people cured of HD and destined to live for several decades. It is, therefore, important to ask how the risks can be minimized.

Information concerning total doses, fractionation and overall treatment time has accumulated sufficiently that a much improved therapeutic ratio can be expected. There is a rather steep dose-response relationship for the most serious consequences of radiation therapy for HD. If only the major intermediate term (6 months to 3 years) consequences of radiation myelopathy, symptomatic pneumonitis and pericarditis are included (fig. 3) [22], it is evident

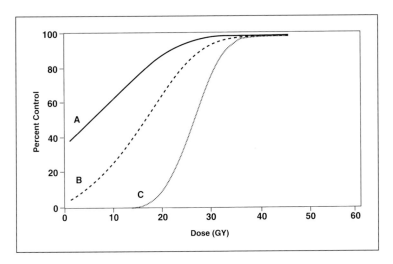

Fig. 4. Dose response for tumor control by tumor size: A = subclinical, B = clinical <6 cm, C = >6 cm nodes. (Reprinted with permission from Vijayakumar and Myriantho-poulos [28].)

that total doses in excess of 40 Gy especially if delivered with fractions of 2.0 Gy or larger, increase the risk of adverse effects.

The dose-response relationship for control of HD is sigmoid as is the case with other tissues and tumors. Estimates of the total dose required to control overt manifestations of HD have evolved slowly over the past three decades. Although the total doses required might seem quite modest relative to the doses required to control common epithelial malignant tumors, the volume irradiated with irregular fields in HD and the wide variety of normal tissues encompassed magnifies the risks. A retrospective review [23] of a large body of data from the literature led to a recommendation to use at least 40 Gy and perhaps as much as 44 Gy to insure consistent control. Reanalysis of these data [24] presented as a sigmoid function of total dose led to a downward revision of recommendation for the total dose required closer to 30 Gy. Data from individual [25, 26] and the Patterns of Care Studies (PCS) [27] corroborated the adequacy of total doses between 33 and 38 Gy and suggested that fractions of 1.5–1.8 Gy were as effective as larger-sized fractions. A thorough reanalysis of available data in the literature was presented by Vijayakumar and Myrianthopoulos [28] in 1992. They identified 4,117 anatomic sites at risk for recurrence after radiation therapy for HD and evaluated them as a function of the size of the tumor (fig. 4). They concluded that a 98% probability of control was achievable with a total dose of 32.4 Gy for subclinical disease,

36.9 Gy for palpable tumors <6 cm in greatest dimension, and 37.4 Gy for tumors >6 cm. The dose-response curves plateaued above those levels such that little gain could be expected with higher total doses. Of course, a much greater risk of normal tissue damage would be anticipated. Brincker and Bentzen [29] suggested that the best-fitting dose-response curves to the data compiled by Vijayakumar and Myrianthopoulos [28] resulted in a plateau at 32.5 Gy and that elapsed time up to 7 weeks had no deleterious effect on local control. More recent PCS reports [30] showed that national practice in the USA had changed little between 1973 and 1983 with respect to total doses used for clinically evident tumors (median 40 vs. 39.9 Gy, respectively); however, the doses administered to clinically uninvolved regions decreased from 40 to 36 Gy.

With all this information, it is possible to devise a treatment approach that carries a high probability of success and a low probability of complications. Total doses of 32.4 Gy for subclinical disease and 37.8 Gy for gross disease, delivered at 1.8 Gy/fraction, seem sufficient. It might be possible to decrease even to 30.6 and 36 Gy, respectively. Indeed, if Brincker and Bentzen [29] are correct in their estimates, 32.4 Gy may be sufficient for all but the most voluminous masses.

Radiation Therapy after Chemotherapy

As might be expected from the preceding discussion, the combination of chemotherapy and radiation therapy must carry increased risks for any and all of the eventualities of treatment. There is no doubt that maximal chemotherapy followed by STNI increases the risks of second malignant tumors, cardiac, pulmonary and gastrointestinal toxicity. Among the possible ways to avoid such effects are elimination of one or the other modality. As noted above, the avoidance of chemotherapy is possible in patients with favorable stage I and II HD.

Is it possible to avoid radiation therapy entirely in patients with unfavorable stage II and stages III and IV? Long-term results of the original MOPP experience from the National Cancer Institute [31] have shown that combination chemotherapy can achieve complete responses in 80% of patients with advanced HD, and approximately 70% of those with complete responses remain free of recurrence 10 years after cessation of all treatment: thus, long-term disease-free survival is achieved in approximately 55% of all patients treated. The most likely sites of failure in patients treated with chemotherapy are those in which disease was clinically evident, especially if bulky. Prosnitz et al. [32] from Yale reported higher disease-free survival rates when combination chemotherapy was followed by radiation therapy to sites of original bulk disease with even lower total doses of irradiation than those recommended above. In children, concerns about irradiation of developing organs, especially bone growth, led to the use of still lower doses to involved fields, namely 15 Gy for children 5 years or less, 20 Gy for children 6–10 years and 25 Gy for those 11–14 years of age [33].

Second Cancer and Treatment of HD

There has been considerable controversy concerning the relative contributions of radiation therapy and chemotherapy to second malignant tumors in patients treated for HD. It is not possible to resolve the issues completely even with the large body of data that has become available in the past 10 years due to a major uncertainty, namely the baseline with which the risk of second cancer must be compared. One baseline is the cancer risk for an age- and sex-matched population in the country of treatment. However, the expected risk cannot be generalized from the USA to Europe as a whole, let alone specific countries within Europe [34] and the age-specific risks may vary even more. Most importantly, the baseline risk of patients with HD alone is not known. Review of a few publications will illustrate the point.

The experience collected through the efforts of a large number of investigators [35] resulted in data from 14,702 patients with HD treated from early 1960s to 1987, is representative of North America and Europe. The cumulative incidence of second cancer rises at the rate of 1% per year among patients who survived at least 1 year after treatment. The cumulative incidence by initial treatment is shown in figure 5. The relative contributions of treatment selection by stage and treatment for relapse, let alone the baseline incidence of second cancer for patients with HD per se, cannot be evaluated.

Rodriguez et al. [36] reported more mature data from the M.D. Anderson Cancer Center concerning the consequences of more intensive chemotherapy when used as the sole modality. They found the hazard ratio for acute myelocytic leukemia (AML) to be 7.3-fold greater for patients who received chemotherapy alone (CT) compared with radiation therapy (RT)±CT. Hazard ratios were 2.4-fold greater for non-Hodgkin's lymphoma (NHL) and 2.1-fold greater for solid tumors with CT alone. Mauch et al. [37] reported the absolute excess risk per 10,000 person-years of AML to be 24.9 for RT+CT vs. 3.6 for RT; corresponding figures for NHL were 10.6 vs. 16.1 and for solid tumors they were 83.9 vs. 36.2. Hancock and Hoppe [38] used relative risk (observed/expected) for comparison of treatments. Although there were striking increases in the risk of AML when CT was used, there was relatively little difference

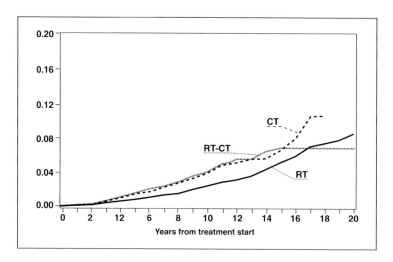

Fig. 5. Cumulative incidence of second cancer-related death by initial treatment in patients who achieved complete remission (radiation therapy (RT)=5,799 patients; chemotherapy alone (CT)=2,201 patients; radiation therapy plus chemotherapy (RT-CT)=4,283 patients). (Reprinted with permission from HenryAmar [37].)

in NHL (RT=29.6, RT+CT=44.5, CT=22.8) and solid tumors (RT=4.3, RT+CT=4.6, CT=2.5).

To what degree are the second solid tumors related to the radiation therapy and to what degree they might be lessened by decreasing the dose-fractionation parameters are unclear. In a long-term outcome experience [39] of 145 patients with stage I HD from MDACC, with a median follow-up of 16.5 years, 15 second malignant tumors were found: 6 were outside the fields of irradiation. This emphasizes the uncertainty of the baseline expectations for risk of second cancer in HD.

Conclusions

Medical decisions must always be made on the basis of more fragmentary information than one would wish. An interpretation of the information presented above has led to the following recommendations for patients at The University of Texas M.D. Anderson Cancer Center. Laparotomy has been abandoned as unnecessarily invasive, fraught with risk of morbidity and mortality and not associated with improved outcome. STNI alone is used in favorable patients with supradiaphragmatic stage I and II HD. Total doses are limited to 30.6 Gy for subclinical disease and a maximum of 39.6 Gy to bulk disease at 1.8 Gy/fraction. In patients who are otherwise favorable, but have large mediastinal masses, 3 cycles of chemotherapy with mitoxantrone (Novantrone), vincristine (Oncovin), vinblastine and prednisone [40] are used to shrink the mediastinal mass to permit protection of the lung, followed by STNI. Patients with unfavorable features (B symptoms, elevated β_2-microglobulin, ESR > 50, 4 or more nodal regions involved, age > 50 years) received 6 cycles of ABVD followed by involved field radiation to sites of original bulk disease. If there is a complete clinical and radiological response, total doses between 25.2 and 30.6 Gy are used depending upon the original size of the mass. If there is a partial response, involved field radiation therapy is used with a total dose of 39.6 Gy at 1.8 Gy/fraction. It is our hypothesis that this treatment plan walks the fine line between high probability of success and low probability of late sequelae.

References

1   Moore CV: Diseases of the reticuloendothelial system; in Cecil RL, Loeb RF, Gutman AB, McDermott W, Wolff HG (eds): A Textbook of Medicine, ed 10. Philadelphia, Saunders, 1959, pp 1095–1105.
2   Ries LAG, Miller BA, Hankey BF, Kosary CL, Harras A, Edwards BK: SEER Cancer Statistics Review, 1973–1991: Tables and Graphs. NIH Publ No 94-2789. Bethesda, National Cancer Institute, 1994.
3   Gilbert R, Babaiantz L: Notre méthode de rœntgenthérapie de la lymphogranulomatose (Hodgkin): Résultats éloignés. Acta Radiol Oncol 1931;12:523–529.
4   Peters MV, Middlemiss KCH: A study of Hodgkin's disease treated by irradiation. Am J Roentgenol Radiat Ther Nucl Med 1958;79:114–121.
5   A Collaborative Study: Survival and complications of radiotherapy following involved and extended field therapy of Hodgkin's disease: Stages I and II. Cancer 1976;38:288–305.
6   Rosenberg SA, Kaplan HS, Hoppe RT, Kushlan P, Horning S: The Stanford randomized trials of the treatment of Hodgkin's disease 1967–1980; in Rosenberg SA, Kaplan HS (eds): Malignant Lymphomas: Etiology, Immunology, Pathology, Treatment. New York, Academic Press, 1982, pp 513–522.
7   De Vita VT, Serpick AA, Carbone PP: Combination chemotherapy in the treatment of advanced Hodgkin's disease. Ann Intern Med 1970;73:891–895.
8   Longo DL, Young RC, Wesley M, Hubbard SM, Duffey PL, Jaffe ES, DeVita VT: Twenty years of MOPP chemotherapy for Hodgkin's disease. J Clin Oncol 1986;4:1295–1306.
9   Santoro A, Bonadonna G: Prolonged disease-free survival in MOPP-resistant Hodgkin's disease after treatment with Adriamycin, bleomycin, vinblastine and dacarbazine (ABVD). Cancer Chemotherapy Pharmacol 1979;2:101–105.
10 Glatstein E, Trueblood HW, Enright LP, Rosenberg SA, Kaplan HS: Surgical staging of abdominal involvement in unselected patients with Hodgkin's disease. Radiology 1970;97:425.
11 Carbone PP, Kaplan HS, Musshoff K, Smithers DW, Tubiana M: Report of the Committee on Hodgkin's Disease Staging Classification. Cancer Res 1971;31:1860–1861.
12 Cox JD: Lymphomas and leukemia; in Cox JD (ed): Moss' Radiation Oncology: Rationale, Technique, Results. St Louis, Mosby-Year Book, 1994, vol 7, pp 795–826.
13 Castellino RA: Imaging techniques for staging abdominal Hodgkin's disease. Cancer Treat Rep 1982;66:697–700.
14 Marglin S, Castellino R: Lymphographic accuracy in 632 consecutive, previously untreated cases of Hodgkin's disease and non-Hodgkin's lymphoma. Radiology 1981;140:351–353.

15   Mendenhall NP: Diagnostic procedures and guidelines for the evaluation and follow-up of Hodgkin's disease. Semin Oncol 1996;6:131–145.
16   Tubiana M, Hayat M, Henry-Amar M, Breur K, van der Werf-Messing B, Burgers M: Five-year results of the EORTC randomized study of splenectomy and spleen irradiation in clinical stage I and II of Hodgkin's disease. Eur J Cancer 1981;17:355–363.
17   Carde P, Hagenbeek A, Hayat M, Monconduit M, Thomas J, Burgers MJV, Noordijk EV, Tanguy A, Meerwaldt JH, Le Fur R, Sommers R, Kluin-Nelemans HC, Busson A, Breed WP, Bron D, Holdrinet A, Rutten EHJM, Michiels JJ, Regnier R, Debusscher L, Musella R, Fargeot P, Thyss A, Cattan A, Rigal-Huguet F, Roth S, Caillou B, Dupouy N, Henry-Amar M: Clinical staging versus laparotomy and combined modality with MOPP versus ABVD in early-stage Hodgkin's disease: The H6 twin randomized trials from the European Organization for Research and Treatment of Cancer Lymphoma Cooperative Group. J Clin Oncol 1993;11:2258–2272.
18   Cox JD, Stoffel TJ: Clinical versus pathologic stage I and II Hodgkin's disease. Oncology 1980;37: 325–328.
19   Tate DJ, Hoppe RT: Pelvic relapse following subtotal lymphoid irradiation in early stage Hodgkin's disease – An analysis of risk, management, and outcome. Int J Radiat Oncol Biol Phys 1995;32: 1239–1244.
20   Noordijk EM, Carde P, Mandard A-M, Mellink WAM, Monconduit M, Eghbali H, Tirelli U, Thomas J, Somers R, Dupouy N, Henry-Amar M: Preliminary results of the EORTC-GPMC controlled clinical trial H7 in early-stage Hodgkin's disease. Ann Oncol 1994;5(suppl 2):107–112.
21   Lacher MJ, Redman JR: Hodgkin's Disease: The Consequences of Survival. Philadelphia, Lea & Febiger, 1990.
22   Fazekas JT, Cox JD, Turner M: Irradiation of stage I and II Hodgkin's disease. Am J Roentgenol Radiat Ther Nucl Med 1975;123:154–162.
23   Kaplan HS: Evidence for a tumoricidal dose level in the radiotherapy of Hodgkin's disease. Cancer Res 1966;26:1221–1224.
24   Fletcher GH, Shukovsky LJ: The interplay of radiocurability and tolerance in the irradiation of human cancers. J Radiol Electrol Med Nucl 1975;56:383–400.
25   Thar TL, Million RR, Hausner RJ, McKetty MH: Hodgkin's disease, stages I and II: Relationship of recurrence to size of disease, radiation dose, and number of sites involved. Cancer 1979;43:1101–1105.
26   Schewe KL, Reavis J, Kun LE, Cox JD: Total dose, fraction size and tumor volume in the local control of Hodgkin's disease. Int J Radiat Oncol Biol Phys 1988;15:25–28.
27   Hanks GE, Kinzie JJ, White RL, Herring DF, Kramer S: Patterns of care outcome studies: Results of the National Practice in Hodgkin's Disease. Cancer 1983;51:569–573.
28   Vijayakumar S, Myrianthopoulos LC: An updated dose-response analysis in Hodgkin's disease. Radiother Oncol 1992;24:1–13.
29   Brincker H, Bentzen SM: A re-analysis of available dose-response and time-dose data in Hodgkin's disease. Radiother Oncol 1994;30:227–230.
30   Hoppe RT, Hanlon AL, Hanks GE, Owen JB: Progress in the treatment of Hodgkin's disease in the United States, 1973 versus 1983. Cancer 1994;74:3198–3203.
31   DeVita VT: The consequences of the chemotherapy of Hodgkin's disease: The 10th David A. Karnofsky Memorial Lecture. Cancer 1981;47:1–13.
32   Prosnitz LR, Farber LR, Kapp DS, Bertino JR, Nordluna M, Lawrence R: Combined modality therapy for advanced Hodgkin's disease: Long-term follow-up data. Cancer Treat Rep 1982;66: 871–879.
33   Donaldson SS, Link MP: Combined modality treatment with low-dose radiation and MOPP chemo-therapy for children with Hodgkin's disease. J Clin Oncol 1987;5:742–749.
34   Parker SL, Tong T, Bolden S, Wingo PA: Cancer statistics, 1997. CA Cancer J Clin 1997;47:5–27.
35   Henry-Amar M: Workshop statistical report; in Somers R, Henry-Amar M, Meerwaldt JK, Carde P (eds): Treatment Strategy in Hodgkin's Disease. Colloques INSERM, vol 196. Paris, Libbey, 1990, pp 169–418.
36   Rodriguez MA, Fuller LM, Zimmerman SO, Allen PK, Brown BW, Munsell MF, Hagemeister FB, McLaughlin P, Velasquez WS, Swan FJ, Cabanillas FF: Hodgkin's disease: Study of treatment intensities and incidences of second malignancies. Ann Oncol 1993;4:125–131.

37   Mauch PM, Kalish LA, Marcus KC, Coleman CN, Shulman LN, Krill E, Come S, Silver B, Canellos GP, Tarbell NJ: Second malignancies after treatment for laparotomy staged IA-IIIB Hodgkin's disease: Long-term analysis of risk factors and outcome. Blood 1996;9:3625–3632.

38   Hancock SL, Hoppe RT: Long-term complications of treatment and causes of mortality after Hodgkin's disease. Semin Radiat Oncol 1996;6:131–145.

39   Vlachaki M, Ha CS: Hagemeister FB, Fuller LM, Rodriguez MA, Besa PC, Hess MA, Brown B, Cabanillas F, Cox JD: Long-term outcome of treatment for Ann Arbor stage I Hodgkin's disease: Patterns of failure, late toxicity and second malignancies. Int J Radiat Oncol Biol Phys 1997;39: 609–616.

40   Hagemeister FB, Cabanillas F, Velasquez WS, Meistrich ML, Liang JC, McLaughlin P, Redman JR, Romaguera JE, Rodriguez MA, Swan F Jr, Fuller LM: NOVP: A novel chemotherapeutic regimen with minimal toxicity for treatment of Hodgkin's disease. Semin Radiat Oncol 1990;17: 34–40.

James D. Cox, MD, Department of Radiation Oncology – Box 97, The University of Texas
M.D. Anderson Cancer Center, 1515 Holcombe Boulevard, Houston, TX 77030 (USA)

Meyer JL (ed): Radiation Injury. Advances in Management and Prevention.
Front Radiat Ther Oncol. Basel, Karger, 1999, vol 32, pp 98–109

....
Hyperbaric Therapy for Radiation Injury

Paul Cianci

Department of Hyperbaric Medicine, Doctors Medical Center, San Pablo, Calif. and
John Muir Medical Center, Walnut Creek, Calif., USA

Background

Hyperbaric oxygen therapy is the intermittent administration of 100%
oxygen at pressure greater than sea level. The technique may be implemented
in a walk-in (multiplace) chamber, compressed to depth with air, in which the
patient breathes 100% oxygen through a mask, head tent, or endotracheal
tube. Alternatively, the patient may be treated in a monoplace (one-person)
chamber pressurized with 100% oxygen. In either case, the arterial partial
pressure of oxygen will approach 1,500 mm Hg at a pressure equivalent of
33 ft of seawater. Hyperbaric oxygen therapy is the primary treatment for
decompression sickness (the bends) and arterial gas embolism [1]. It has been
demonstrated a useful adjunct in the treatment of clostridial myonecrosis
[2–5], severe carbon monoxide poisoning [6–12], soft and hard tissue radiation
damage [13–20], necrotizing anaerobic infections [21, 22], crush injury [23–27],
chronic refractory osteomyelitis [28], compartment syndrome, and compromised flaps or grafts [29–34]. Some centers are utilizing this modality in the
treatment of acute thermal injury [35–42].

During the 1930s, oxygen at pressure was proposed as a treatment for
decompression sickness [43]. In the early 60s, Dutch investigators showed the
efficacy of hyperbaric oxygen in the treatment of gas gangrene and anemic
states [44, 45]. Later in that decade it became the standard therapy for US
Naval diving casualties [46]. Subsequent studies have shown the importance
of oxygen in the treatment of problem wounds [35–37, 47], enhancement of
white cell killing ability [48], preservation of compromised tissue [49] and
angiogenesis [13, 50–52]. The clinical indications for the use of hyperbaric
oxygen as an adjunct continue to be expanded and defined.

Mechanism of Action

Oxygen inhaled at pressure dissolves in plasma. At 3 atm an arterial PO_2 of nearly 2,200 may be achieved. Up to 6.9 vol% of oxygen may be forced into solution, a quantity sufficient to maintain life in the absence of hemoglobin [45].

Fibroblast Proliferation

Abnormally low tissue PO_2 will result in stimulation of fibroblast activity. Many nonhealing tissues are hypoxic, i.e. tissue oxygen tensions are frequently in the range of 5–15 mm Hg. Tissue oxygen tensions of 30–40 mm Hg, however, are necessary for fibroblast turnover, collagen synthesis, and the development of a collagen matrix for capillary ingress into avascular areas. This can be accomplished through the intact circulation with adjunctive hyperbaric oxygen therapy [53, 54].

Neovascularization

Restoration of abnormally low tissue PO_2 levels to physiologic values will result in capillary proliferation. The previously stimulated fibroblasts serve as a matrix and support for new capillary growth.

Enhancement of White Cell Killing

Polymorphonuclear cells in low oxygen tensions (e.g. 5–15 mm Hg) show diminished ability to kill organisms through the peroxidase system, an oxygen-dependent mechanism [55]. The killing ability of white cells can be greatly enhanced as oxygen tensions increase [48, 56–58].

Vasoconstriction

Exposure to oxygen at pressure causes a 20% reduction in blood flow, resulting in less diapedesis and bleeding in areas of capillary damage and a reduction of edema. The tenfold increase in oxygen content of plasma more than compensates for decreased arterial flow.

Toxicity and Side Effects

Risks involved in the use of hyperbaric oxygen therapy are related to pressure changes and the toxic effects of oxygen. They include barotrauma to the ears or sinuses, pulmonary overpressure accidents with pneumothorax, grand mal seizures, and pulmonary toxicity. Trauma to the ears or sinuses may be averted with slow compression, the use of decongestants, and patient education. Occasionally ear squeezes may necessitate the insertion of temporary pharyngiotympanic tubes [59]. Pulmonary trauma is a more serious occurrence. Careful pretreatment evaluation for pulmonary blebs or air trapping due to bronchospasm or secretions is mandatory. An additional minor side effect is a change in visual acuity which occurs after approximately 20 treatments. This is a transient phenomenon and is unassociated with any demonstrable pathology. There is no evidence that protocols currently used in the United States as recommended by the Undersea and Hyperbaric Medical Society cause cataracts. Oxygen toxicity represents a special problem. Oxygen is a drug with definite dose-related complications and side effects related to depth and duration of treatment. Two well-recognized problems deserve comment.

Oxygen Seizures

Susceptibility to oxygen-induced grand mal seizures is subject to individual variance. As PO_2 increases, so does the risk of oxygen-induced seizures. For this reason, oxygen treatment is limited to a maximum of 3 atm absolute (equivalent to 66 ft of seawater in depth) in all human exposures. Fever and certain medications also predispose to this complication. The risk of oxygen seizures is particularly enhanced by elevated arterial pressure of carbon dioxide. Drugs that suppress respiration are therefore likely to increase the risk of oxygen toxicity when they are used during the hyperbaric therapy. Agents such as narcotics and sedatives must be used cautiously. Oxygen seizures are rare and usually self-limited, responding to the cessation of oxygen breathing.

Pulmonary Toxicity

Damage to lung manifested by a decrease in vital capacity and irritation to the large airways is a predictable complication of prolonged oxygen exposure at depth [60]. For this reason, treatment protocols are designed to minimize oxygen toxicity and to utilize the shallowest depth consistent with desired results. These complications of oxygen therapy can be avoided by intermittent exposure and are, in fact, relatively rare.

Claustrophobia

Confinement anxiety may be a problem for a small percentage of patients. This is particularly true in the smaller, monoplace chambers. Sedation and reassurance will usually remedy the problem, but some patients are not able to tolerate treatment despite these measures.

Clinical Applications

Currently accepted conditions as recommended by the Undersea and Hyperbaric Medical Society include gas embolism, carbon monoxide poisoning, crush injury and acute traumatic ischemia, decompression sickness, gas gangrene, necrotizing soft tissue infections, osteomyelitis (refractory), radiation necrosis, osteoradionecrosis and soft tissue radiation injury, compromised skin grafts and flaps, enhancement of healing in selected problem wounds, and thermal burns [61]. The rationale for treatment of decompression sickness and arterial gas embolism, whether due to diving accidents or iatrogenically induced, as might occur in a lung biopsy or vascular procedure, is the compression and counterdiffusion of bubbles and hyperoxygenation of compromised tissue. Treatment in a recompression chamber is mandatory for either of these entities. Treatment of severe carbon monoxide poisoning is based on the knowledge that hyperbaric oxygen hastens carboxyhemoglobin dissociation, reverses hypoxia, and may antagonize lipid peroxidation. Mortality and morbidity are favorably influenced by its use.

Radiation necrosis, soft tissue radiation injury, and osteoradionecrosis share a common pathophysiology of obliterative endarteritis with resultant tissue ischemia and hypoxia. Daily elevation of hypoxic tissue PO_2s to normal or supranormal levels results in development of a functioning capillary bed through which planned surgery can be accomplished. Unplanned but required surgery in previously irradiated tissue was fraught with a high incidence of potentially fatal complications. Adjunctive hyperbaric oxygen therapy is indicated in the postoperative state in this clinical setting. A coordinated program of adjunctive hyperbaric oxygen therapy now constitutes the most successful and cost-effective method of dealing with these difficult problems.

The work of Marx et al. in defining the true nature of the biologic injury has been helpful in understanding how hyperbaric oxygen can be of value in the treatment of this difficult problem. His triad of hypovascularity, hypocellularity and hypoxia serves as a matrix for utilization of this useful clinical tool and was elegantly described in the National Cancer Institute Monograph Consensus Statement No. 9, 1990 [62]. This discussion will attempt to provide an overview of the problem, specifically addressing the significant contributions and advances in therapy utilizing adjunctive hyperbaric oxygen therapy in the comprehensive management of such patients.

Recent data suggest that hyperfractionation can significantly reduce the rate of complications from radiation therapy [63]. There remains, however, a significant number of patients that suffer the complications of radiation therapy, including bone necrosis and soft tissue damage. Many of these perplexing clinical problems can be helped by the judicious use of adjunctive hyperbaric oxygen therapy as part of an aggressive program involving plastic repair and newer surgical techniques.

The use of hyperbaric oxygen in the treatment of radiation damage dates to the early 70s and the work of Mainous and co-workers [64–66]. By 1977, Tobey et al. [67] had suggested that favorable response was dose-related. By the late 70s, Farmer et al. [68] and Davis et al. [69] had reported significant healing utilizing hyperbaric oxygen as an adjunctive treatment for radiation necrosis of soft and hard tissue. In the late 70s and early 80s, a clearer definition of the nature of the injury and its response to intermittent elevation of oxygen tensions emerged [70–72]. In 1983, Marx [72] reported a high success rate in 58 patients treated with aggressive surgery and adjunctive hyperbaric oxygen therapy. By 1988, he had accumulated a large experience showing a high rate of success utilizing a staging protocol and carefully timed surgery [20]. He demonstrated via transcutaneous oxygen measurements that capillary density in previously irradiated tissue was improved to approximately 80% of normal over time, and this effect was durable (fig. 1) [62].

This aggressive approach based on sound understanding of physiologic principles has resulted in an economical approach to the difficult problem of head and neck radiation damage. Marx's initial report in 1984 demonstrated the cost-effectiveness of the aggressive Marx/University of Miami protocol. Bringing these to 1995 dollars, he showed that surgery without hyperbaric oxygen support resulted in an 8% success rate, a USD 38,000 per year cost, and USD 140,000 lifetime cost. Hyperbaric oxygen without surgery resulted in a 17% success rate, a USD 16,000 per year cost, and a USD 83,000 lifetime cost. The Marx/Miami protocol resulted in a 92% resolution for a USD 44,000 full one-time cost [73]. It would thus appear that this approach to the difficult problem of head and neck radiation damage is justified.

Prevention of osteonecrosis in a previously irradiated field when tooth extraction is necessary is best served by 20 treatments prior to extraction and 10 treatments postoperatively, this approach being based on a randomized prospective clinical trial in 74 patients. The incidence of osteonecrosis in patients not receiving preventive hyperbaric oxygen therapy was 29 vs. 5.4% in the treated group [73].

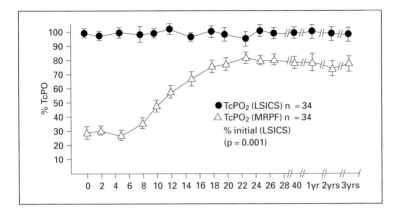

Fig. 1. Changes in vascular density (measured by transcutaneous oxygen (TcPO₂) record-ings at the left intercostal space (LSICS) and at the center of the irradiated area (MRPF)) of irradiated tissue as a function of hyperbaric oxygen exposures. Horizontal scale is marked in months and years. p = 0.001 for irradiated vs. nonirradiated tissue. [From 62, with permission.]

Bony or soft tissue reconstruction in an area of prior radiation is fraught with danger [66, 74–77]. Work by Johnson and Marx has shown a high rate of success and a lower complication rate in 407 boney reconstructions; and in 160 patients randomized to HBO or non-HBO therapy, wound dehiscence occurred in 8% of the HBO-treated patients vs. 48% in the non-HBO group, infection was 6 and 24%, respectively, and defective wound healing was noted in 11 vs. 55%. Marx has also demonstrated in an elegant study [78, 79] the relationship of oxygen dose to angiogenesis. He subjected irradiated rabbits to a course of adjunctive hyperbaric oxygen therapy. There was a clear and statistically highly significant relationship between the dose of oxygen rendered and the degree of angiogenesis noted (fig. 2) [50]. An accompanying editorial comment stated 'This is a nicely performed study; the data are clean, and the conclusions are supported. It is of more biologic than practical surgical use since radiation is seldom administered in doses that interfere with surgery and hyperbaric oxygen therapy is not a practical way of treating most patients with irradiation effects' [50]. The reader is left to his own conclusions.

Recent Developments

Recently, a greater appreciation of the value of adjunctive hyperbaric oxygen therapy in soft tissue radiation damage has evolved. Williams et al. [80] described in a prospective, observational study, 14 patients with necrotic

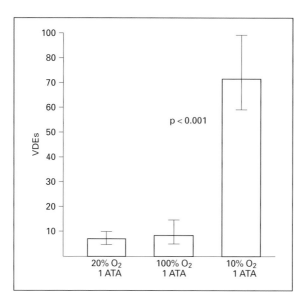

Fig. 2. VDE measurements versus partial pressures of O_2 graph identifying an increased vascular density of the hyperbaric oxygen group over the normobaric oxygen group and the normobaric air group. [From 50, with permission.]

wounds of the pelvis which had failed to improve with conservative therapy. Outcome was resolution of necrosis. Fourteen patients underwent 15 courses of hyperbaric oxygen treatment. Sight of the cancer was cervix in 9, endometrium in 1, vagina in 3, and colon in 1. Mean radiation dose was 4,830 cGy. Fifty-three percent had additional intracavatary radiation. Thirteen patients had complete resolution; 1 patient did not resolve. The editors pointed out that the study took 5 years to obtain 14 patients. All had failed conventional therapy. Their prospects included progressive disability, addiction and death. The editors stated 'The value of careful observation by seasoned clinicians is established'. Feldmeier et al. [81] have reported 9 severe laryngeal necroses cases treated with hyperbaric oxygen therapy. In this group, there were no laryngectomies, 3 previously trachyectomized patients were decannulated, 2 fistulae closed spontaneously, and 2 were closed surgically; there were no permanent hyperbaric complications. Feldmeier's group [82] has additionally reported 23 cases of delayed radiation injury of the chest wall. In this report, 6 of 8 soft tissue injuries healed; of 15 boney involvements, 8 resolved with aggressive treatment, 3 patients had residual tumor present, and there was a 60% overall resolution rate. In a subsequent report, this same group reported 41 patients suffering from delayed radiation injury of the abdomen and/or pelvis [83]. Twenty-six healed, 6 showed healing failure, 9 received an inadequate course of hyperbaric oxygen therapy, and overall, success rate was 81%.

Radiation cystitis deserves special consideration. There have been numerous reports of successful management of hemorrhagic cystitis and radiation injury of the bladder [84–88]. Most recently, Bevers et al. [89] reported 40 patients in a prospective study who received 20 sessions of 100% oxygen at 3 atm for 90 min. All patients had biopsy-proven radiation cystitis and severe hematuria. Hematuria disappeared completely or improved markedly in 37 patients after treatment. Mean follow-up was 23 months, with a recurrence rate of 0.12 per year. There were no adverse effects.

The efficacy of adjunctive hyperbaric oxygen therapy for the treatment of radiation complications in children has been discussed by Ashamalla et al. [90]. In a series of 10 patients who had received high doses of radiation, there was a 90% favorable response.

Future Directions

The utilization of adjunctive hyperbaric oxygen therapy in other areas is presently being studied. Larsen et al. [91] showed improved osseous integration of implants into previously irradiated bone. The HBO-treated animals showed better histologic integration at 10 and 16 weeks; better soft tissue healing was observed. The author suggested that further animal and clinical studies were warranted. Warren and Cianci [92] recently reported the treatment of chronic radiation proctitis. In 14 patients, 8 had complete resolution, 1 had substantial improvement, and 5 were nonresponders. The overall success rate was 64%, with a 17-month follow-up. Feldmeier et al. [93] studied the effect of early intervention for the prevention of bowel injury. Thirty hyperbaric treatments were rendered 7 weeks after radiation in an animal model. Hyperbaric oxygen resulted in less bowel rigidity and less narrowing ($p < 0.007$). The authors suggested that further studies, including human trials, were warranted.

There is concern that hyperbaric oxygen could have a cancer-promoting effect. In a review of 24 reports, 12 clinical, 11 animal, and 1 both, Feldmeier et al. [94] showed 3 positive and 10 negative in the human studies, 2 positive and 10 negative in the animal studies, and concluded that the literature failed to support cancer enhancement by hyperbaric oxygen therapy.

In summary, the use of adjunctive hyperbaric oxygen therapy in carefully selected cases can ameliorate the difficult problems of dealing with hard and soft tissue radiation damage. The relative safety of the treatment and the excellent results obtained, particularly as part of an aggressive combined team approach, militate for its consideration in the treatment of radiation injury.

References

1 Davis JC, Elliot DH: Treatment of the decompression disorders; in Bennet PB, Elliot DH (eds): The Physiology and Medicine of Diving, ed 3. San Pedro, Best Publisher, 1982, pp 473–486.
2 Heimbach RD: Gas gangrene: Review and update. Hyperbar Oxygen Rev 1980;1:41–61.
3 Hart GB, Lamb RC, Strauss MB: Gas gangrene. I. A collective review. J Trauma 1983;23:991–995.
4 Hart GB, Lamb RC, Strauss MB: Gas gangrene. II. A 15-year experience with hyperbaric oxygen. J Trauma 1983;23:995–1000.
5 Bakker DJ: Pure and mixed aerobic and anaerobic soft tissue infections. Hyperbar Oxygen Rev 1985;6:65–96.
6 Goulon M, Barios A, Rapin M: Carbon monoxide poisoning and acute anoxia due to breathing coal gas and hydrocarbons. Ann Méd Interne (Paris) 1969;120:335–349/J Hyperbar Med 1986;1: 23–41.
7 Myers RAM, Snyder SK, Linberg S, Cowley RA: Value of hyperbaric oxygen in suspected carbon monoxide poisoning. JAMA 1981;246:2478–2480.
8 Myers RAM, Snyder SK, Emhoff TA: Subacute sequelae of carbon monoxide poisoning. Ann Emerg Med 1985;14:1163–1167.
9 Ziser A, Shupak A, Halpern P: Delayed hyperbaric oxygen treatment for acute carbon monoxide poisoning. Br Med J 1984;289:960.
10 Yee IM, Brandon GK: Successful reversal of presumed carbon monoxide induced semicoma. Aviat Space Environ Med 1983;54:641–643.
11 Norkool DM, Kirkpatrick JN: Treatment of acute carbon monoxide poisoning with hyperbaric oxygen: A review of 115 cases. Ann Emerg Med 1985;14:1168–1171.
12 Mathieu D, Nolf M, Durocher A, Saulnier F: Acute carbon monoxide poisoning risk of late sequelae and treatment by hyperbaric oxygen. Clin Toxicol 1985;23:315–324.
13 Marx RE: Osteoradionecrosis of the jaws: Review and update. Hyperbar Oxygen Rev 1984;5:48–126.
14 Marx RE: A new concept in the treatment of osteoradionecrosis. J Oral Maxillofac Surg 1983;41: 351–357.
15 Mainous EG, Boyne PJ, Hart GB, Terry BC: Restoration of resected mandible by grafting with combination of mandible homograft and autogenous iliac marrow and postoperative treatment with hyperbaric oxygen. J Oral Surg 1973;35:13–20.
16 Mainous EG, Hart GB: Osteoradionecrosis of the mandible: Treatment with hyperbaric oxygen. Arch Otolaryngol Head Neck Surg 1975;101:173–177.
17 Mainous EG, Boyne PJ: Hyperbaric oxygen in total rehabilitation of patients with mandibular osteoradionecrosis. J Oral Maxillofac Surg 1974;3:197–201.
18 Marx RE, Ames JR: The use of hyperbaric oxygen therapy in bony reconstruction of the irradiated and tissue deficient patient. J Oral Maxillofac Sur 1982;40:412–420.
19 Marx RE, Johnson RP, Kline SN: Prevention of osteoradionecrosis: A randomized prospective clinical trial of hyperbaric oxygen vs. penicillin. J Am Dent Assoc 1985;111:49–54.
20 Marx RE, Johnson RP: Problem wounds in oral and maxillofacial surgery: The role of hyperbaric oxygen; in Davis JC, Hunt TK (eds): Problem Wounds: The Role of Oxygen. New York, Elsevier, 1988, pp 65–123.
21 Riseman JA, Zamboni WA, Curtis A, Graham DR, Konrad HR, Ross DS: Hyperbaric oxygen therapy for necrotizing fasciitis reduces mortality and the need for debridements. Surgery 1990;108: 847–850.
22 Gozal D, Ziser A, Shupak A, Ariel A, Melamed Y: Necrotizing fasciitis. Arch Surg 1986;121: 233–235.
23 Schramek A, Hashmonai M: Vascular injuries in the extremities in battle casualties. Br J Surg 1977; 64:644–648.
24 Shupak A, Gozal D, Ariel A, Melamed Y, Katz A: Hyperbaric oxygenation in acute peripheral post-traumatic ischemia. J Hyperbar Med 1987;2:7–14.
25 Strauss MB, Hart GB: Crush injury and the role of hyperbaric oxygen. Top Emerg Med 1984;6:9–24.
26 Nylander G, Lewis D, Nordstrom H, Larsson J: Reduction of post-ischemic edema with hyperbaric oxygen. Plast Reconstr Surg 1985;76:596–601.

27   Nylander G, Lewis D, Nordstrom H, Larsson J: Metabolic effects of hyperbaric oxygen in post-ischemic muscle. Plast Reconstr Surg 1987;79:91–96.

28   Strauss MB: Chronic refractory osteomyelitis: Review and role of hyperbaric oxygen. Hyperbar Oxygen Rev 1980;1:231–255.

29   Tan CM, Im MJ, Myers RAM, Hoopes JE: Effects of hyperbaric oxygen and hyperbaric air on the survival of island skin flaps. Plast Reconstr Surg 1984;73:27–30.

30   Nemiroff PM, Merwin GE, Brant T, Cassisi NJ: Effects of hyperbaric oxygen and irradiation on experimental flaps in rats. Otolaryngol Head Neck Surg 1985;93:485–491.

31   Nemiroff PM, Merwin GE, Brant T, Cassisi NJ: HBO and irradiation on experimental skin flaps in rats. Surg Forum 1984;35:549–550.

32   Nemiroff PM, Lungu AL: The influence of hyperbaric oxygen and irradiation on vascularity in skin flaps: A controlled study. Surg Forum 1987;38:565–567.

33   Perrins DJD: Hyperbaric oxygenation of skin flaps. Br J Plast Surg 1966;19:440.

34   Kaelin CM, Im MJ, Myers RAM, Manson PN, Hoopes JE: The effects of hyperbaric oxygen on free flaps in rats. Arch Surg 1990;125:607–609.

35   Cianci P, Petrone G, Drager S, Lueders H, Lee H, Shapiro R: Salvage of the problem wound and potential amputation with wound care and adjunctive hyperbaric oxygen therapy: An economic analysis. J Hyperbar Med 1988;3:127–141.

36   Cianci P, Lueders H, Lee H, Shapiro R, Green B, Williams C: Hyperbaric oxygen and burn fluid requirements: Observations in 16 patients with 40–80% TBSA burns. Undersea Biomed Res Suppl 1988;15:14.

37   Cianci P, Lueders H, Lee H, Shapiro R, Sexton J, Williams C, Green B: Adjunctive hyperbaric oxygen reduces the need for surgery in 40–80% burns. J Hyperbar Med 1988;3:97–101.

38   Cianci P, Lueders HW, Lee H, Shapiro RL, Sexton J, Williams C, Sato R: Adjunctive hyperbaric oxygen therapy reduces length of hospitalization in thermal burns. J Burn Care Rehabil 1989;10: 432–435.

39   Cianci P: Personal survey, 1990.

40   Cianci P, Williams C, Lueders H, Lee H, Shapiro R, Sexton J, Sato R: Adjunctive hyperbaric oxygen in the treatment of thermal burns – An economic analysis. J Burn Care Rehabil 1990;11:140–143.

41   Grossman AR, Grossman AJ: Update on hyperbaric oxygen and treatment of burns. Hyperbar Oxygen Rev 1982;3:51–59.

42   Hart GB, O'Reilly RR, Broussard ND, Cave RH, Goodman DB, Yanda RL: Treatment of burns with hyperbaric oxygen. Surg Gynecol Obstet 1974;139:693–696.

43   Yarbrough OB, Behnke AR: The treatment of compressed air illness utilizing oxygen. J Ind Hyg Toxicol 1939;21:6.

44   Brummelkamp WH, Hoogendiji J, Boerema I: Treatment of anaerobic infections (clostridial myositis) by drenching the tissues with oxygen under high atmospheric pressure. Surgery 1961;49:299–302.

45   Boerema I, Meijne NG, Brummelkamp WH, Bouma S, Mensch MH, Kamermans F, Hanf S, Van Aalderen A: Life without blood: A study of the influence of high atmospheric pressure and hypothermia on dilution of blood. J Cardiovasc Surg 1960;1:133–146.

46   Goodman MW, Workman RP: Oxygen-breathing approach of treatment of decompression sickness in divers and aviators. Bureau of Medicine and Surgery. BuShips Project SF0110606, Task 11513-2, Research Report 5-65, 1965.

47   Davis JC: Hyperbaric oxygen therapy. J Intens Care Med 1989;4:55–57.

48   Mader JT, Brown GL, Guckian JC, Wells CH, Reinarz JA: A mechanism for the amelioration of hyperbaric oxygen of experimental staphylococcal osteomyelitis in rabbits. J Infect Dis 1980;142: 915–922.

49   Baroni G, Porro T, Faglia E, Pizzi G, Mastropasqua M, Oriani G, Pedesini G, Favales F: Hyperbaric oxygen in diabetic gangrene treatment. Diabetes Care 1987;10:81–86.

50   Marx RE, Ehler WJ, Tayapongsak P, Pierce LW: Relationship of oxygen dose to angiogenesis induction in irradiated tissue. Am J Surg 1990;160:519–524.

51   Sheffield PJ: Tissue oxygen measurement with respect to soft tissue wound healing with normobaric and hyperbaric oxygen. Hyperbar Oxygen Rev 1985;6:18–46.

52   Sheffield PJ, Dunn JM: Continuous monitoring of tissue oxygen tension during hyperbaric oxygen therapy; in Smith G (ed): Proceedings of the Sixth International Congress on Hyperbaric Medicine. Aberdeen, University Press, 1977, pp 125–129.

53   Pai MP, Hunt TK: Effect of varying oxygen tensions on healing of open wounds. Surg Gynecol Obstet 1972;135:756–758.

54   Niinikoski J: Effect of oxygen supply on wound healing and formation of experimental granulation tissue. Acta Physiol Scand Suppl 1969;1:334.

55   Hohn DC, MacKay RD, Halliday B, Hunt TK: Effect of oxygen tension on the microbial function of leukocytes in wounds and in vitro. Surg Forum 1976;27:18–20.

56   Hunt TK: The physiology of wound healing. Ann Emerg Med 1988;17:1265–1273.

57   Knighton DR, Halliday B, Hunt TK: Oxygen as an antibiotic: The effect of inspired oxygen on infection. Arch Surg 1984;119:199–204.

58   Rabkin J, Hunt TK: Infection and oxygen; in Davis JC, Hunt TK (eds): Problem Wounds: The Role of Oxygen. New York, Elsevier, 1988, pp 1–16.

59   Ross JC, Cianci PE: Barotitis media resulting from hyperbaric oxygen therapy. A retrospective study of 395 consecutive cases. Undersea Biomed Res Suppl 1990;17:102.

60   Clark JM, Fisher AB: Oxygen toxicity and extension of tolerance in oxygen therapy; in Davis JC, Hunt TK (eds): Hyperbaric Oxygen Therapy. Bethesda, Undersea Medical Society, 1977, pp 61–67.

61   Hyperbaric Oxygen Therapy: A Committee Report. Kensington, Undersea and Hyperbaric Medical Society, 1996.

62   Myers RAM, Marx RE: Use of hyperbaric oxygen in postradiation head and neck surgery; in Fox PC, Janson CC (eds): National Cancer Institute Monographs, No 9. Bethesda, National Institutes of Health, 1990, pp 151–157.

63   Garden AS, Morrison WH, Ang KK, Peters LJ: Hyperfractionated radiation in the treatment of squamous cell carcinomas of the head and neck: A comparison of two fractionation schedules. Int J Radiat Oncol Biol Phys 1995;31:493–502.

64   Mainous EG, Boyne PJ, Hart GB: Elimination of sequestrum and healing of osteoradionecrosis of the mandible after hyperbaric oxygen therapy: Report of a case. J Oral Surg 1973;31:336.

65   Mainous EG, Boyne PJ: Hyperbaric oxygen in the total rehabilitation of patients with mandibular osteoradionecrosis. Int J Oral Surg 1974;3:297–302.

66   Hart GB, Mainous EG: The treatment of radiation necrosis with hyperbaric oxygen. Cancer 1976; 37:2580–2585.

67   Tobey RE, Kelly JF, Vinton JR, Baker RD: Hyperbaric oxygen therapy for chronic osteoradionecrosis of the mandible; in Smith G (ed): Proceedings of the Sixth International Congress on Hyperbaric Medicine. Aberdeen, University Press, 1977, pp 1–275.

68   Farmer JC, Shelton DL, Bennett PD, Angelillo JD, Hudson WR: Treatment of radiation-induced tissue injury by hyperbaric oxygen. Ann Otol Rhin Laryngol 1978;87:707–715.

69   Davis JC, Dunn JM, Gates GA, Heimbach RD: Hyperbaric oxygen – A new adjunct in the management of radiation necrosis. Arch Otolaryngol 1979;105:58–61.

70   Marx RE, Johnson RP: Studies in the radiobiology of osteoradionecrosis and their clinical significance. Oral Surg 1978;64:379–390.

71   Beehner MR, Marx RE: Hyperbaric oxygen-induced angiogenesis and fibroplasia in human irradiated tissues; in Proceedings of the 65th Meeting of the American Association of Oral and Maxillofacial Surgery, 1983, pp 78–79.

72   Marx RE: Osteoradionecrosis: A new concept of its pathophysiology. J Oral Maxillofac Surg 1983; 41:283–288.

73   Marx RE: Radiation injury to tissue; in Kindwall EP (ed): Hyperbaric Medicine Practice. Flagstaff, Best Publishing, 1994, pp 447–503.

74   Ariyan S, Krizek TJ: Radiation effects: Biological and surgical considerations; in McCarthy JD (ed): Plastic Surgery. Philadelphia, Saunders, 1990, pp 831–848.

75   Robinson DW: Surgical problems in the excision and repair of radiated tissue. Plast Reconstr Surg 1975;55:41.

76   Rudolph R: Complications in surgery for radiotherapy skin damage. Plast Reconstr Surg 1982;70: 179–185.

77   Joseph DL, Shumrick DL: Risks of head and neck surgery in previously irradiated patients. Arch Otolaryngol 1973;97:381–384.

78   Marx RE, Johnson RP: Clinical and pathophysiological studies in oral surgery. Presented at Clinical Management of Problem Wounds, San Antonio, April 25–28, 1991.

79   Marx RE, Johnson RP: Studies in the radiobiology of osteoradionecrosis and their clinical significance. Oral Surg Oral Med Oral Pathol 1987;64:379–390.

80   Williams JA, Clarke D, Dennis W, Dennis EJ, Smith ST: The treatment of pelvic soft tissue radiation necrosis with hyperbaric oxygen. Am J Obstet Gynecol 1992;167:412–416.

81   Feldmeier JJ, Heimbach RD, Davolt DA, Brakora MJ: Hyperbaric oxygen as an adjunctive treatment for severe laryngeal necrosis: A report of nine consecutive cases. Undersea Hyperbar Med 1993; 20:329–335.

82   Feldmeier JJ, Heimbach RD, Davolt DA, Court WS, Stegmann BJ, Sheffield PJ: Hyperbaric oxygen as an adjunctive treatment for delayed radiation injury of the chest wall: A retrospective review of twenty-three cases. Undersea Hyperbar Med 1995;22:383–393.

83   Feldmeier JJ, Heimbach RD, Davolt DA, Court WS, Stegmann BJ, Sheffield PH: Hyperbaric oxygen an adjunctive treatment for delayed radiation injuries of the abdomen and pelvis. Undersea Hyperbar Med 1996;23:205–213.

84   Weiss JP, Mattei DM, Neville EC, Hanno PM: Primary treatment of radiation-induced hemorrhagic cystitis with hyperbaric oxygen: 10-year experience. J Urol 1994;151:1514–1517.

85   Weiss JP, Boland FP, Mori H, Gallagher M, Brereton H, Preate DL, Neville EC: Treatment of radiation-induced cystitis with hyperbaric oxygen. J Urol 1985;134:352–354.

86   Norkool DM, Hampson NB, Gibbons RP, Weissman RM: Hyperbaric oxygen therapy for radiation-induced hemorrhagic cystitis. J Urol 1993;150:332–334.

87   Schoenrock GJ, Cianci P: Treatment of radiation cystitis with hyperbaric oxygen. Urology 1986; 27:271–272.

88   Lee HC, Liu CS, Chiao C, Lin SN: Hyperbaric oxygen therapy in hemorrhagic radiation cystitis: A report of 20 cases. Undersea Hyperbar Med 1994;21:321–327.

89   Bevers RFM, Bakker DJ, Kurth KH: Hyperbaric oxygen treatment for haemorrhagic radiation cystitis. Lancet 1995;346:803–805.

90   Ashmalla HL, Thom SR, Goldwein JW: Hyperbaric oxygen therapy for the treatment of radiation-induced sequelae in children. Cancer 1996;77:2407–2412.

91   Larsen PE, Stronczek MJ, Beck FM, Rohrer M: Osteointegration of implants in radiated bone with and without adjunctive hyperbaric oxygen. J Oral Maxillofac Surg 1993;51:280–287.

92   Warren DC, Cianci PE: Chronic radiation proctitis treated with hyperbaric oxygen. Presented at Winter Symposium on Baromedicine, Snowbird, January 14–17, 1996.

93   Feldmeier JJ, Jelen I, Davolt DA, Valente PT, Meltz ML, Alecu R: Hyperbaric oxygen as a prophylaxis for radiation-induced delayed enteropathy. Radiat Oncol 1995;35:138–144.

94   Feldmeier JJ, Heimbach RD, Davolt DA, Brakora MJ, Sheffield PJ, Porter AT: Does hyperbaric oxygen have a cancer-causing or -promoting effect? A review of the pertinent literature. Undersea Hyperbar Med 1994;21:467–475.

Paul Cianci, MD, Department of Hyperbaric Medicine, Doctors Medical Center,
San Pablo, CA 94806, and John Muir Medical Center, Walnut Creek, CA (USA)

Meyer JL (ed): Radiation Injury. Advances in Management and Prevention.
Front Radiat Ther Oncol. Basel, Karger, 1999, vol 32, pp 110–119

....

Gastrointestinal Toxicity of Infusional Chemoradiation

Tyvin A. Rich

Department of Radiation Oncology, University of Virginia Health Sciences Center,
Charlottesville, Va., USA

Introduction

Chemotherapy given with external beam irradiation (chemoradiation) for cancers of the gastrointestinal (GI) tract has been studied for several decades. 5-Fluorouracil (5-FU) has been the mainstay since it is the single most active agent in GI cancers and it is a radiation sensitizer. 5-FU given as an infusion during irradiation in phase III trials for cancers of the esophagus [1], rectum [2], and the anal canal [3] is superior to irradiation alone thus validating its role in the management of these malignant diseases. From these and other studies has emerged data suggesting ways to reduce both the acute and late morbidity of combined modality therapy based on the administration schedule of the radiosensitizing chemotherapy with concurrent irradiation. Reviewed here are various chemoradiation trials with emphasis on acute and late toxicity of combined modality therapy. One interpretation of these data strongly suggests that *fractionation of both modalities* in a course of chemoradiation may widen the therapeutic window.

5-FU: A Time-Dependent Drug

A wide variety of chemotherapeutic agents have been used with irradiation but this review will focus exclusively on the antimetabolite 5-FU. The basic mechanisms of action of 5-FU are well understood and have been reviewed elsewhere [4]; it is one of few agents that has been evaluated in GI cancer patients in a wide range of doses, schedules, and methods of administration.

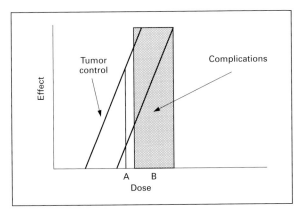

Fig. 1. Dose-response curves for rate invariant (A) versus high-dose (B) administration of an antineoplastic agent with a short half-life. The shaded box represents a range of drug concentrations for a dose administration schedule where the agent is given by rapid bolus administration. The resulting high toxicity is associated with the high initial drug levels that typically occur (5-FU is a good example). The rapid fall in drug concentration may then produce less toxicity and have continued cytotoxicity, but because of these wide variations in concentration this technique of radiosensitizer administration is less able to split the therapeutic window compared to the method depicted by A. With rate invariant radiosensitizer administration the therapeutic window can be split better.

For GI chemoradiation the protracted venous infusional (PVI) schedule of 5-FU has become increasingly popular and is based on translational research indicating 5-FU to be more cytotoxic when given by prolonged exposure in vitro [5]. Another preclinical observation is that the use of prolonged exposure removes the variability of response of human cancers to this agent when compared to short acute exposures [6].

The scientific validation of the clinical utility of PVI 5-FU compared to a bolus administration schedule is based largely on phase III data in patients with metastatic colorectal cancer [7]. In another way, practical clinical validation has considered the differences in the administration schedules of 5-FU have had on the therapeutic window. In the case where the chemotherapy is delivered with a rate invariant system, the therapeutic window can be widened by either increased antitumor activity and altered normal tissue toxicity [8]. Depending on the method of administration of the radio-sensitizing 5-FU chemoradiation there is the potential for less severe toxicity by PVI compared to bolus 5-FU chemoradiation since the dosage is administered in a constant fashion which eliminates the drug peaks associated with unacceptable systemic toxicity (fig. 1).

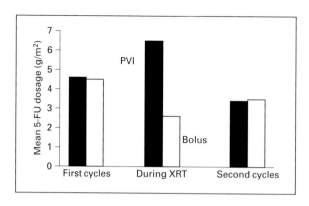

Fig. 2. A histogram of the total 5-FU doses delivered in a rectal adjuvant trial comparing protracted venous infusion to (PVI) bolus administration. The higher total PVI dose was associated with less local failure and higher survival for equal (but different type) acute toxicity. The higher total PVI dose was administered over 6–7 weeks compared to the short intermittent dosing of the bolus therapy.

Acute reactions seen with PVI include mucocutaneous reactions and the hand-foot syndrome and less hematologic toxicity than is seen with bolus therapy. Although the cellular mechanisms responsible for these differential phenomena remain elusive, prolonged exposure to cytotoxic chemotherapy mimics a form of fractionation. The use of small daily doses of chemoradiotherapy may also parallel observations from the radiotherapy clinic that fractionation spares late effects.

Based on the observations of the superior effect of 5-FU PVI in metastatic colorectal cancer and on a pilot study of PVI chemoradiation [9], 5-FU PVI chemoradiation was compared to bolus 5-FU chemoradiation in the adjuvant treatment of patients with stage II and III rectal cancer [2]. PVI 5-FU chemoradiation improved local control (p = 0.08) and significantly improved disease-free and overall survival (p ≤ 0.05) with roughly equal toxicity rates in each arm, although there was a preponderance of mucocutaneous toxicity in the PVI arm. One explanation for these differences is shown in figure 2 where the total doses of 5-FU have been plotted for each course according to treatment arm. The histogram shows that the delivered doses of 5-FU during the systemic phases were identical but the total doses during irradiation were 2–3 times higher in the PVI compared to the bolus arm. The higher total doses in the 'fractionated' PVI 5-FU arm are higher because of the dose-sparing when the drug is given slowly.

Rich

Chemoradiation: A Form of Accelerated Treatment

Irradiation schedules using multiple daily X-ray doses have permitted the delivery of total doses over relatively short periods and is referred to as accelerated radiotherapy [10]. One rationale for this approach is to overcome the effect of cancer cell proliferation that creates a need for higher total doses (up to 2–3 Gy/week) in the treatment of a variety of cancers [11]. With chemoradiation a similar analogy exists where the additional daily dose is given with systemic cytotoxic therapy instead of a second irradiation dose. Chemoradiation can be evaluated in terms of the pattern of dose application (fractionation) now firmly rooted in an understanding of cellular radiobiology. In spite of our limited knowledge of the mechanisms of action of chemotherapy and irradiation, clinical treatment programs are largely empiric descriptions of the therapeutic window. Radiation oncologists have long used the dose-effect curves to interpret results of radiotherapy schedules and this approach is used here for the interpretation of the results of combined modality therapy. The advantages of delivering a chemotherapy dose in this case with rate invariant methods splits a narrow therapeutic window and there is the suggestion that further widening can be achieved with fractionation. Central to this evaluation is the assessment of early and late reactions (occurring in rapidly and slowly proliferating tissues) after irradiation alone compared to those occurring after infusional chemoradiation therapy. The clinical infusional 5-FU chemoradiation schedules that have been studied are the short, high-intensity delivery of 5-FU for 4–5 days (at a dosage of 1,000 mg/m^2 [12], or protracted schedules using continuously 5-FU for 30–60 days (at dosages of 200–300 mg/m^2) [13]. Some of the main infusional 5-FU chemoradiation schedules that have been used are illustrated for comparison in figure 3.

Another reason for the increasing use of 5-FU and other drugs with infusional chemoradiation techniques is the convenience of ambulatory therapy by using portable pumps which are widely available at reasonable cost. In addition, the availability of safe vascular access, obtained with a variety of intravenous catheters, has also fostered this treatment approach in the outpatient setting.

Several human cancer sites will be used to illustrate the similarities of chemoradiation to accelerated therapy. In the treatment of head and neck cancer it has recently been shown that there is a therapeutic advantage for the use of treatment schedules that shortens overall time of irradiation when compared to a conventional treatment course [14]. With accelerated irradiation the main treatment effects are a shorter latent time to onset and greater level of acute effects compared to conventional treatment [15]. Similarly, there is a similar finding with the use of combined modality therapy where the second

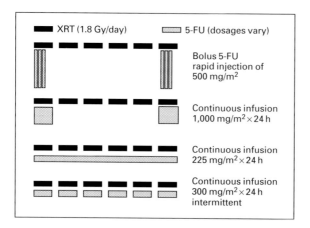

Fig. 3. A comparison of different 5-FU infusional schedules used in the treatment of GI malignancies. XRT schedules shown are typically given 9 Gy/week for a total of 5–6 weeks. The height of the 5-FU box is proportional to the peak serum concentrations that are achieved with different treatment schedules. The use of PVI schedules avoids the serum peaks and valleys of drug concentration associated with acute toxicity as depicted in figure 1.

daily treatment is 5-FU chemotherapy instead of radiotherapy which results in a statistically significant shorter time to onset and a greater severity of acute reactions compared to irradiation alone for head and neck cancer [16].

In the treatment of esophageal cancer, a recent randomized trial has shown that the use of infusional chemoradiation is superior to irradiation alone [1]. There are increased acute toxicities as well as increased late normal tissue toxicities (table 1).

In anal canal cancer, chemoradiation is now the standard management since the results with conservation treatment are equivalent to surgery and this combination of treatment can preserve organ function in the majority of cases. Chemoradiation not only improves local control but it also achieves better survival when compared to historical surgical controls. Recent phase II [17, 18] and III [19] chemoradiation trials indicate that colostomy-free survival is achieved in about 75% and overall survival rate at 5 years is ~70–75%. The use of infusional 5-FU with mitomycin or cisplatin appears to be better than single-agent 5-FU chemoradiation [20]. In the RTOG randomized trial, both 5-FU and mitomycin radiation sensitization (FUMIR) was most effective in stage T3 and T4 anal canal cancers and in those with histologically proven inguinal lymph node involvement [19]. Successful control of anal cancer has been associated with acute and late morbidity. In the RTOG trial a 23% grade 3 and 4 toxicity rate occurred in those receiving FUMIR compared to only

Table 1. A comparison of the acute and late morbidity of 5-FU infusional chemoradiation compared to irradiation alone for esophageal cancer patients treated on RTOG-85-01

Toxicity type	65 Gy	50 Gy 5-FU (1,000 mg/m^2) Cisplatin (75 mg/m^2)
Acute	5%	20–30%[1]
Late	19%	22–14%

The increase in acute toxicity is expected with the concurrent administration of S-phase-specific agents that attack the rapidly proliferating cell compartment. The equal late toxicity rate for surviving patients is also surprising since the total radiation dose was 22% less than that used in the irradiation alone arm. A potential way in the future to reduce the late complication rate could be with the use of lower daily doses of radiosensitizing chemotherapy.

[1] Range given for randomized and nonrandomized treatment groups treated with chemoradiation.

7% who received FUIR (5-FU + Irradiation). A comparison of late effects in various chemoradiation protocols in the management of anal canal cancer supporting this hypothesis is shown in table 2. Evidence for similar sparing of late effects with protracted infusional chemoradiation in the rectal adjuvant trial also provides support to this argument. Recent evidence that large daily doses of chemoradiation can increase late effects also comes from the randomized EORTC trial which reported no overall increase in late effects. However, they did report that late effects in only the anus were higher in those treated with chemoradiation compared to those given irradiation alone [3].

Newer Chemoradiation Approaches

Biomolecular studies of 5-FU metabolism have resulted in an understanding of some of the potential control points in the production of toxic intermediates that could be exploited for clinical use. One pathway of 5-FU metabolism that can be manipulated to increase the cytotoxic effect is through the prolongation of the inhibition of thymidylate synthase by the concurrent use of the methyl-group donor leucovorin [21]. Clinical studies with 5-FU combined with leucovorin have shown increased anticancer effects based on the increased rate of response seen in patients treated with this combination

Table 2. A comparison of toxicities reported in the treatment of chemoradiation for anal cancer; there is a suggestion that the use of lower daily dose chemoradiation is associated with lower rates of late complications

Series Ref.	Patients (n)/ randomized	XRT total/ daily dose, Gy	Chemotherapy, dose per m²			Late morbidity Gd 3/4
			5-FU	Mito	cddP	
RTOG 18	79/no	40.8/1.7	1,000 mg (96 h) × 1	10 mg Bolus × 1		17 'late' skin reactions, 2 necrosis, 1 stenosis
RTOG 19	291/yes	45–54/1.8	1,000 mg (96 h) × 2	10 mg Bolus × 2		7 vs. 23% for 5-FU ± mitomycin, respectively[1]
EROTC 3	110/yes	60–65²/1.8	750 mg (96 h) × 2	Bolus × 1		Anal ulcer and fistula: 5 XRT vs. 11 CXRT
MDACC 17	58/no	45–60/1.8	300 mg protracted infusions³		± 4.0 mg	None

[1] Only grade 4 toxicity; includes acute toxicity.
[2] Total doses includes implant boost.
[3] Protracted infusions of both 5-FU and cisplatin.

compared to 5-FU alone [22]. However, in a large randomized study in the adjuvant treatment of operable rectal cancer with this combination as a radiation sensitizer, there was no better outcome with biomodulated 5-FU compared to bolus 5-FU alone [23]. In this same study there was an increased level of normal tissue toxicity for those treated with biomodulated 5-FU (higher hematologic and mucocutaneous toxicity) compared to those receiving only bolus 5-FU. One interpretation of these data is that the biomodulated bolus 5-FU is a relatively large single dose and its use is associated with greater acute injury and potentially increased late effects compared to those seen with fractionated schedules.

Another approach to widen the therapeutic window of 5-FU chemoradiation is to alter the timing of the administration of the radiation sensitizer to coincide with the maximal tolerance of the host [24]. The preclinical basis for circadian 5-FU infusional chemoradiation are the observations that the toxicity of S-phase inhibitors (like 5-FU and other antimetabolites) can be lowered by when the agents are administered [25]. These different toxicity rates are related, in part, to the variation in proliferation rates in the GI tract and the bone marrow which are circadian-dependent; the toxicity of a variety of systemic agents can be altered by selecting a treatment time when there is relatively lower proliferation in these tissues [26]. Another reason for better tolerance is related to the chronopharmacology of 5-FU which is known to have a strong circadian dependency [27]. These preclinical observations have served as the basis of a clinical hypothesis which has been tested in clinical trials with 5-FU-based systemic chemotherapy and shows a therapeutic gain when a circadian schedule was compared to bolus administration [28]. Building onto these clinical data of systemic chemotherapy alone, circadian 5-FU infusional chemoradiation has been reported from the University of Florida where low toxicity was seen in the treatment of patients with T4 rectal cancer [29]. In this trial the relatively low toxicity rate is associated with a 28% complete response rate which for these stages of disease is remarkable. Further trials with this approach are warranted to confirm if the circadian timing of administration is exploitable in other patient populations and for other tumor sites with 5-FU infusional chemoradiation as well as with other newer agents.

For GI cancers, the use of radiation dose fraction size of 1.8–2.0 Gy is based on the tumor control rates obtained at acceptable levels of acute and late morbidity. New treatment planning techniques that can assess normal tissue volumes, along with newer planning methods to obtain optimal dose distributions for the cancer volume, will achieve better sparing of the normal tissues. One treatment technique that had been extensively studied is the belly board or the open tabletop which allows the movement of the small intestine away from the pelvis so that the posterior pelvis can be treated while sparing the more anteriorly located small bowel. This method or some other small bowel exclusion technique should be employed in the treatment of the posterior pelvis. Assessment of late damage should not be limited to the assessment of just grade 4 toxicity that requires a reoperation for small bowel obstruction. Newer quality-of-life tools are available and need to be integrated into the management of patients with gastrointestinal cancers. Education of the patient about the basic facts of the anatomy and how their GI tract functions are important but simple tools that can sometimes make important differences for patients. Another important management issue is the use of fluids and fiber after treatment.

Infusional chemoradiation programs will likely increase because there is evidence that this approach is valuable and that there are different types and severity of toxicities compared to conventional bolus administration schedules. The best method is still not known but building onto the knowledge base of what had been described in the last several decades with the use of irradiation alone, the use of a fractionated approach for both irradiation and chemotherapy is one that appears to spare normal tissue damage.

References

1   Herskovic A, Martz K, al-Sarraf M, Leichman L, Brindle J, Vaitkevicius V, Cooper J, Byhardt R, Davis L, Emami B: Combined chemotherapy and radiotherapy compared with radiotherapy alone in patients with cancer of the esophagus [see comments]. N Engl J Med 1992;326:1593–1598.

2   O'Connell MJ, Martenson JA, Wieand HS, Krook JE, Macdonald JS, Haller D, Mayer RJ, Gunderson LL, Rich TA: Improving adjuvant therapy for rectal cancer by combining protracted-infusion fluorouracil with radiation therapy after curative surgery. N Engl J Med 1994;331:502–507.

3   Bartelink H, Roelofsen F, Eschwege F, Rougier P, Bosset JF, Gonzales D, Peiffert D, van Glabbeke M, Pierart M: Concomitant radiotherapy and chemotherapy is superior to radiotherapy alone in the treatment of locally advanced anal canal cancer: Results of a phase III randomized trial of the European Organization for Research and Treatment of Cancer Radiotherapy and Gastrointestinal Cooperative Groups. J Clin Oncol 1997;15:2040–2049.

4   Pu T, Robertson JM, Lawrence TS: Current status of radiation sensitization by fluorinated pyrimidines. Oncology 1995;9:707–735.

5   Smalley SR, Kimler BF, Evans RG, Dalziel WC: Heterogeneity of 5-fluorouracil radiosensitivity modulation in cultured mammalian cell lines. Int J Radiat Oncol Biol Phys 1992;24:519–525.

6   Byfield JE, Calabro-Jones P, Klisak I, Kulhanian F: Pharmacologic requirements for obtaining sensitization of human tumor cells in vitro to combined 5-fluorouracil or ftorafur and X-rays. Int J Radiat Oncol Biol Phys 1982;8:1923–1933.

7   Lockich JJ, Ahlgren JD, Gullo JJ, Philips J, Fryer J: A prospective randomized comparison of continuous infusion fluorouracil with a conventional bolus schedule in metastatic colorectal carcinoma: A Mid-Atlantic Oncology Program Study. J Clin Oncol 1989;7:425–432.

8   Goldman P: Rate-controlled drug delivery. N Engl J Med 1982;29:286–290.

9   Rich TA, Lokich JJ, Chaffey JT: A pilot study of protracted venous infusion of 5-fluorouracil and concomitant radiation therapy. J Clin Oncol 1985;3:402–406.

10 Peters LJ: Accelerated fractionation using the concomitant boost: A contribution of radiobiology to radiotherapy. BJR Suppl 1992;24:200–203.

11 Fowler JF, Lindstrom MJ: Loss of local control with prolongation in radiotherapy. Int J Radiat Oncol Biol Phys 1992;23:457–467.

12 Byfield JE: The clinical use of 5-fluorouracil and other halopyrimidines as radiosensitizers in man; in Lokich J (ed): Cancer Chemotherapy by Infusion. Chicago, Precept Press, 1987, pp 479–501.

13 Rich TA: Chemoradiation for gastrointestinal cancer; in Vaeth JM, Meyer JL (eds): Front Radiat Ther Oncol. Basel, Karger, 1992, pp 115–130.

14 Horiot JC, Begg AC, Le Fur R, Schraub S, van den Bogaert W, van Glabbeke M, Pierart M: Present status of EORTC trials of hyperfractionated and accelerated radiotherapy on head and neck carcinoma. Recent Results Cancer Res 1994;134:111–119.

15 Thames HD, Bentzen SM, Turesson I, Overgaard M, Van den Bogaert W: Time-dose factors in radiothaerapy: A review of the human data. Radiother Oncol 1990;19:219–235.

16 Browman GP, Cripps C, Hodson I, Eapen L, Sathya L, Levine MN: Placebo-controlled randomized trial of infusional fluorouracil during standard radiotherapy and locally advanced head and neck cancer. J Clin Oncol 1994;12:2648.

17 Rich TA, Ajani JA, Morrison WH, Ota D, Levin B: Chemoradiation therapy for anal cancer: Radiation plus continuous infusion of 5-fluorouracil with or without cisplatin. Radiother Oncol 1993;27:209–215.

18 Sischy B, Doggett RLS, Krall JM, Taylor DG, Sause WT, Lipsett JA, Seydel G: Definitive irradiation and chemotherapy for radiosensitization in management of anal carcinoma: Interim report on RTOG study 83-14. J Natl Cancer Inst 1989;81:850–856.

19 Flam M, John M, Pajak TF, Petrelli N, Myerson R, Doggett S, Quivey J, Rotman M, Kerman H, Coia L, Murray K: Role of mitomycin in combination with fluorouracil and radiotherapy, and of salvage chemoradiation in the definitive nonsurgical treatment of epidermoid carcinoma of the anal canal: Results of a phase III randomized intergroup study. J Clin Oncol 1996;14:2527–2539.

20 Cummings BJ: Anal canal carcinomas; in Front Radiat Ther Oncol. Basel, Karger, 1992, vol 26, pp 131–141.

21   Zhang ZG, Harstrick A, Rustum YM: Modulation of fluoropyrimidines: Role of dose and schedule of leucovorin administration. Semin Oncol 1992;19(suppl 3):10–15.

22   Erchlichman C, Fine S, Wong A, Elhakim T: A randomized trial of fluorouracil and folinic acid in patients with metastatic colorectal cancer. J Clin Oncol 1988;6:469–475.

23   Tepper JE, O'Connell MJ, Petroni GR, Hollis D, Cooke E, Benson AB III, Cummings B, Gunderson LL, Macdonald JS, Martenson JA: Adjuvant postoperative fluorouracil-modulated chemotherapy combined with pelvic radiation therapy for rectal cancer: Initial results of intergroup 0114. J Clin Oncol 1997;15:2030–2039.

24   Halberg F, Halberg J, Halberg E, Halberg F: Chronobiology, radiobiology, and steps toward the timing of cancer radiotherapy; in Cancer Management in Man: Detection, Diagnosis, Surgery, Radiology, Chronobiology, Endocrine Therapy. Dordrecht, Kluwer Academic, 1989, p 227.

25   Bjarnason GA, Hrushesky WJM: Cancer chronotherapy; in Hrushesky WJM (ed): Circadian Cancer Therapy. Boca Raton, CRC Press, 1994, p 241–263.

26   Sheving LE, Sheving LA, McClellan JL, Feners RJ: Experimental basis for circadian cancer chemotherapy. J Infus Chemother 1995;5:3–7.

27   Zhang R, Diasio R: Pharmacologic basis of circadian pharmacodynamics; in Hrushesky WJM (ed): Circadian Cancer Therapy. Boca Raton, CRC Press, 1994, pp 61–103.

28   Levi FA, Zidani R, Vannetzel J-M et al: Chronomodulated versus fixed-infusion-rate delivery of ambulatory chemotherapy with oxaliplatin, fluorouracil, and folinic acid (leucovorin) in patients with colorectal cancer metastasis: A randomized multi-institutional trial. J Natl Cancer Inst 1994; 86:1608–1617.

29   De W, Marsh R, Chu N-M, Vauthey J-N, Mendenhall WM, Lauwers GY, Bewsher C, Copeland E: Preoperative treatment of patients with locally advanced unresectable rectal adenocarcinoma utilizing continuous chronobiologically shaped 5-fluorouracil infusion and radiation therapy. Cancer 1996;78:217–225.

Tyvin A. Rich, MD, Department of Radiation Oncology, Box 383,
University of Virginia Health Sciences Center, Charlottesville, VA 22903 (USA)

Meyer JL (ed): Radiation Injury. Advances in Management and Prevention.
Front Radiat Ther Oncol. Basel, Karger, 1999, vol 32, pp 120–126

....

Management of Radiation-Induced Urologic Complications

Harcharan Gill

Division of Urology, Stanford University, Stanford, Calif., USA

Radiation injury to the urinary tract can occur either from the direct treatment of a malignancy of the urinary tract (bladder, prostate) or from treatment of adjacent organs (cervix, uterus, ovary). Urologic complications are classified as early or late, with early complications occurring during or immediately after treatment. Late complications develop many months to years after treatment and are due to reaction in the vascular, connective and parenchymal tissue. Urologic complications are divided into mild, moderate and severe depending on the symptoms and this often helps in planning the treatment required to resolve the complication [1–10].

The majority of the urologic complications occur in the lower urinary tract. These result from treatment of the prostate, bladder, rectum, cervix and uterus. Upper urinary tract complications can occur following treatment of the retroperitoneum, and kidneys. Most major complications occur late in the course of treatment. The incidence and severity of complications is also dependent on the dose and technique of radiation. In addition there are specific risk factors that predispose a patient to some complications, e.g. incontinence in patients with previous transurethral resection of the prostate (TURP). This section will only address the management of the late complications which include: (1) hemorrhagic cystitis; (2) urinary incontinence; (3) ureteral strictures, and (4) erectile dysfunction.

Hemorrhagic Cystitis

Hemorrhagic cystitis secondary to radiation is an acute or insidious diffuse bleeding from the bladder mucosa. It may be accompanied by dysuria, urgency,

Table 1. Classification to help plan treatment

Mild	No drop in hematocrit, controlled by simple outpatient procedures
Moderate	Hemorrhage producing a progressive drop in hematocrit, requiring less than 6 units of blood
Severe	Hematuria refractory to irrigation, installations, requires more than 6 units of blood

Table 2. Treatment options for each category

Mild	If no clots, observe and increase fluid intake If persistent, oral estrogens or aminocaproic acid If clots, place Foley catheter and irrigate clots and consider oral agents
Moderate	Admit to hospital and irrigate with saline, alum, aminocaproic acid, silver nitrate, or prostaglandin
Severe	Irrigation with formalin under anesthesia Embolization of vesical arteries or open surgery: cystectomy or urinary diversion

urinary frequency and nocturia. The incidence of hemorrhagic cystitis following radiation of pelvic organs is 3–15%. Hematuria may develop months to years after treatment and it may be mild to catastrophic. It is generally not possible to predict patients at risk.

Prevention

Prevention of hemorrhagic cystitis is lacking, and most clinical effort is placed on treatment of established damage. Sodium pentosulfanpolysulfate (Elmiron) is a semisynthetic polyionic compound similar to heparin. It acts by coating the bladder mucosa like the natural glycosaminoglycans. It is given orally, 4–7 weeks after starting treatment. This drug was only recently approved in the USA for interstitial cystitis, and data for radiation cystitis is deficient. In the European literature, Orgotein, a metalloprotein, has been shown to have a preventative role in radiation cystitis when administered intravesically. This drug is not approved in the USA.

Treatment

The management of hemorrhagic cystitis is dependent on the degree of hematuria. Table 1 outlines the classification that helps in planning treatment. Table 2 outlines the specific treatment options for each of the categories. Each

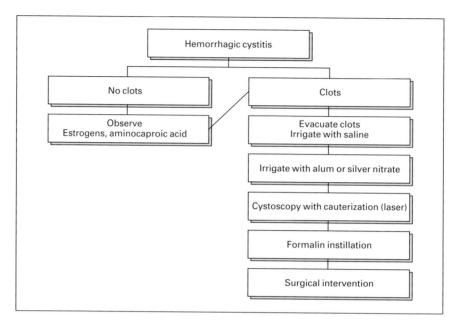

Fig. 1. Algorithm used in the management of hemorrhagic cystitis patients.

of the options is discussed below. An algorithm that I use in the management of these patients is shown in figure 1.

Conservative management: Minor episodes can be treated with urine culture and empiric antibiotics. Patients are instructed to increase oral fluid intake. Oral agents that can be used are estrogens or aminocaproic acid. Conjugated estrogens are used at 1.0–2.0 mg/day. Aminocaproic acid prevents fibrinolysis by inhibiting plasminogen activator substances. A loading oral dose of 5 g is followed by 1 gram orally to a maximum of 30 g in 24 h. The maximal response is achieved within 8–12 h. It is contraindicated in patients suspected to be bleeding from the upper urinary tract.

Evacuation of clots: Irrigate with a large caliber >22-Fr Foley catheter with multiple holes. If this is not successful, consider cystoscopy to evacuate tenacious, organized clots. This can be done under local anesthesia in a clinic. The success of any irrigation depends on the thoroughness of clot evacuation.

Bladder irrigation: A three-way Foley catheter size 22–28 Fr with a 30-cm^3 balloon is used. Saline is run at a rate to keep the efflux clear. Alum and silver nitrate are run at 60–100 cm^3/h.

Cystoscopy: This can be done under local or regional anesthesia. The advantage of doing it under anesthesia is that cauterization of the bleeders can be done at the same time. Electrocautery or Nd:YAG laser are effective in controlling bleeding.

Silver nitrate: A 0.5–1.0% solution in sterile water is used either for instillation or continuous irrigation. This solution has to be protected from light.

Alum: Alum is an ammonium or potassium salt of aluminum in sterile water. 1% solution has a pH of 4.5 and is not absorbed from the bladder. It acts by hardening the capillary endothelium and reduces local edema and inflammation. Serum levels of aluminum should be monitored biweekly to avoid encephalopathy.

Prostaglandin: PGE_2 and PGF_2 are uroprotective when used intravesically. It reduces the mucosal ulceration and improves healing of the microvasculature and epithelium.

Formalin: Act by rapidly fixing the bladder mucosa, thus preventing further blood loss, sloughing and mucosal necrosis. It is painful and thus requires regional or general anesthesia. It is up to 80% effective in refractory bleeding. Instill 50 cm^3 of 1–5% formalin (37% formaldehyde = 100% formalin) for 10 min. A cystogram to rule out vesicoureteral reflux must be done prior to instillation. If reflux is present, ureteral occlusion balloons can be used prior to the instillation to prevent ureteral strictures. Most patients develop small capacity bladder following formalin instillation.

Surgery: If bleeding is progressive despite all the measures outlined above and in the algorithm, surgery should be considered. Percutaneous embolization of the hypogastric artery by the interventional radiologist is helpful for the very ill patient. As an alternative, if the patient's condition allows cystectomy with urinary diversion, this is the most definitive treatment.

Conclusion: The algorithm is merely a guideline for the management of these patients. There are a number of factors that can interfere with the plan of management. These include the patient's general condition, available facilities and the physician's personal experience. The algorithm also guides the patient on the potential options available and to a small degree predicts the expected outcome of the treatment. In my experience, 30% of patients can be successfully managed by outpatient care with antibiotics or other conservative measures. A patient who requires continuous bladder irrigation can be advised that there is a 70% chance that he will not require further hospitalization. Less than 5% of the patients with hemorrhagic cystitis require formalin instillation.

Urinary Incontinence

Urinary incontinence following irradiation of pelvic organs occurs in 1–5% of the patients. Patients with previous prostatic surgery (TURP or radical prostatectomy) are at an increased risk. The pathogenesis of incontinence may be either sphincteric incompetence due to fibrosis, or bladder dysfunction due to a reduced capacity. The former group present with stress incontinence, while patients with bladder problems have predominantly urge incontinence. A small number of patients may have a combination of both bladder and sphincter problems.

Management: It is generally possible from the history to identify the underlying etiology, but in complicated cases urodynamic evaluation by a urologist is necessary. Patients with sphincteric problems are treated with periurethral injection of collagen. This is done as outpatient via a cystoscope and carries a success of 30–50% in the mild group. If this fails, an artificial urinary sphincter is placed. This is a mechanical prosthetic device that is surgically placed around the urethra. Patients should be warned about an increased risk of cuff erosion due to the effects of radiation on the local tissue. The success of an artificial sphincter is 70–80% in patients with normal bladders. If incontinence is due to bladder dysfunction the treatment is pharmacological in mild cases and surgery in severe cases. Anticholinergic and antispasmodics like oxybutinin (Ditropan) at 5 mg 3 times/day are helpful in urge incontinence if the bladder capacity is normal or mildly reduced. In patients with severely reduced bladder capacity, surgery with augmentation cystoplasty using a segment of bowel helps to correct the incontinence. In rare exceptions cystectomy with urinary diversion is necessary to control incontinence.

Erectile Dysfunction

Difficulty with obtaining or maintaining an erection occurs in 5–40% of patients following radiation to bladder or prostate. It can cause significant morbidity to the younger patient, but fortunately a number of therapeutic options are available.

Management: It is seldom necessary to obtain any invasive tests to evaluate erectile dysfunction following radiation. A detailed history and physical exam usually suffices. Three therapeutic options are available:

(1) *Vacuum erection devices*: This mechanical device works to increasing the blood flow into the penis, by creating a vacuum around it. Patient acceptance and satisfaction with these devices range from 60 to 80%.

(2) *Vasoactive agents*: These agents are self-administered either intracavernously or intraurethrally. The former requires self-injection into the penis using a syringe and fine needle. The agents currently available are phentolamine, papaverine and prostaglandin (PGE_1). The transurethral

route became available only recently and is generally more acceptable. Prostaglandin is the only agent marked for this use. The success rate for either of the techniques varies from 60 to 70%.

(3) *Penile prosthesis*: This option is used as a last resort. Malleable or inflatable implants are available and are inserted surgically.

Ureteral Strictures

Ureteral strictures are a late complication of radiation to the cervix, uterus and bladder. The incidence is 1% at 5 years, 2.5% at 20 years with an actuarial risk of 0.15% per year. Patients may present with flank pain, urinary infection and occasionally remain asymptomatic.

Management: A number of options are available, and the least invasive should be tried first. Endoscopic balloon dilatation of the stricture has a 50–60% success in strictures <1.5 cm. If this fails, or the stricture is long, ureteral reimplantation into the bladder is usually successful. A small number of patients are managed with ureteral stents only either due to the underlying medical status or patient preference. These stents have to be changed every 4–6 months. Nephrectomy is the treatment of choice if the kidney is nonfunctioning and the patient is symptomatic.

Conclusion

The long time course of late urological complications suggests the continued surveillance of survivors. Generally the morbidity of most complications is preferable to tumor recurrence. Compromise in the intensity and duration of treatment can result in higher disease recurrence rates. Improved techniques may reduce the incidence in the future. The management of mild complications can be done on an outpatient basis by any health care provider. However, patients with moderate or severe complications should be referred to urologists.

References

1   DeVries CR, Freiha FS: Hemorrhagic cystitis: A review. J Urol 1990;143:1–9.
2   Mukamel E, Lupu A, DeKernion JB: Alum irrigation for severe bladder hemorrhage. J Urol 1986; 135:784–785.
3   Liu YK, Harty JI, Steibbock GS, Holt HJ, Golgstein DA, Amin M: Treatment of radiation or cyclophosphamide induced hemorrhagic cystitis using conjugated estrogen. J Urol 1990;144: 41–43.

4   Dewan AK, Mohan M, Ravi R: Intravesical formalin for hemorrhagic cystitis following irradiation of cancer of the cervix. Int J Gynecol Obstet 1993;42:131–135.
5   Moreno JE, Ahlering TE: Late local complications after definitive radiotherapy for prostatic adenocarcinoma. J Urol 1992;147:926–928.
6   McIntyre JF, Eifel PJ, Levenback C, Oswald MJ: Ureteral strictures as a late complication of radiotherapy for stage 1B carcinomas of the uterine cervix. Cancer 1995;75:836–843.
7   Hart KB, Duclos M, Shamsa F, Forman JD: Potency following conformal neutron/photon irradiation for localized prostate cancer. Int J Radiat Oncol 1996;35:881–884.
8   Conlin MJ, Bagley DH: Incisional treatment of ureteral strictures; in Smith's Textbook of Endourology. St. Louis, Missouri, USA. Quality Medical Publications, 1996, vol 1, pp 497–505.
9   Lue TF: Physiology of erection and pathophysiology of impotence; in Campbell Urology. Philadelphia, Saunders, 1992, vol 1, pp 707–728.
10   Appell RA: Collagen injection therapy for urinary incontinence. Urol Clin North Am 1994;21: 177–178.

Harcharan Gill, MD, Division of Urology S-287, 300 Pasteur Drive, Stanford, CA 94305 (USA)

Meyer JL (ed): Radiation Injury. Advances in Management and Prevention.
Front Radiat Ther Oncol. Basel, Karger, 1999, vol 32, pp 127–144

....

Management of Radiation Effects on the Eye and Orbit

Kathleen B. Gordon, Joan M. O'Brien

Department of Ophthalmology, University of California, San Francisco, Calif., USA

Radiation-induced injury to the eye and ocular adnexa encompasses a wide spectrum of disease, from transient erythema of the eyelid and mild conjunctivitis to corneal perforation and loss of the globe. Not all damage is directly caused by radiation. Injury to one ocular structure may secondarily affect adjacent tissues. For example, damage to the lacrimal gland with resultant dry eye may lead to severe corneal drying, ulceration and perforation of the globe. Although the components of the eye and orbit are discussed separately here, the importance of their interrelationship should be remembered.

Eyelids

Acute radiation-induced changes of the eyelids are usually noted a few days after treatment. Transient skin erythema may develop followed by formation of a crust. The reaction peaks in 10–20 days and usually subsides within 2–4 weeks (fig. 1). Chronic eyelid changes include skin atrophy, cicatricial changes of the skin or conjunctival surface, pallor, telangiectasis and hair loss [1] (fig. 2). Closure of the punctum also has been reported [2] (fig. 3).

Clinical Syndromes
Cicatricial changes of the conjunctival surface may result in an inward rotation of the eyelid margin, or entropion. In cases of entropion, the eyelashes often touch the cornea producing chronic irritation. When chronic, the eyelashes may eventually produce corneal breakdown and scarring. Alternatively, scarring of the eyelid skin may result in an outward rotation of the lid margin, or ectropion (fig. 4). If severe, ectropion results in exposure and drying of the

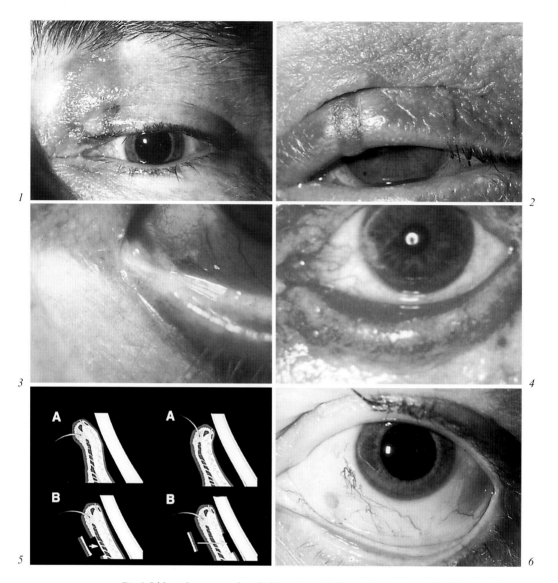

Fig. 1. Lid erythema associated with acute radiation-induced dermatitis. Skin breakdown is seen medially.

Fig. 2. Radiation-associated lash loss. These chronic changes are frequently observed with accelerated particle therapy in cases where the lids cannot be removed from the particle beam.

Fig. 3. Punctal atresia. Chronic changes in the lid margin can result in closure of the puncta with resultant failure of the nasal lacrimal pump system and chronic tearing.

Fig. 4. Primary ectropion. Changes in the lid skin with chronic inflammation following radiation can produce an out-turning of the lid margin known as ectropion.

inferior cornea leading to exposure keratitis. Corneal drying may become so severe as to result in recurrent epithelial breakdown, infection and finally perforation. Though the cornea becomes dry, these patients often complain of chronic tearing because they are unable to pump tears into the nasolacrimal duct normally [1]. The outward turning of the lid results in removal of the puncta from apposition to the tear lake.

Radiation exposure also may cause closure of the puncta, the opening to the nasolacrimal system [2]. Affected patients also complain of chronic tearing. Though eyelid abnormalities may coexist in these patients, the nasolacrimal system should be separately evaluated for patency before a treatment plan is established.

Treatment

Acute skin changes are usually transient and can be treated with lubrication and mild topical steroids as required for patient comfort.

Eyelid malpositions resulting from scarring of either the anterior or posterior lamella with resultant rotation of the lid margin often require surgical correction. Surgery is aimed at restoring the deficient tissue and allowing the eyelid to return to its normal position (fig. 5). In the case of an entropion, the conjunctiva is incised and undermined until freed from the underlying tissue. A cartilage graft, which can be obtained from the ear, is then sutured in between the cut edges. After surgery, the surface epithelializes within 4–6 weeks [3].

Similar principles apply to ectropion repair. A horizontal incision is made along the entire length of the scarred tissue. The skin is then undermined and freed from the underlying orbicularis both superiorly and inferiorly. A skin graft is sewn into place and the eyelids sutured together under tension to prevent excessive shrinkage of the graft. The best color match is usually found in the contralateral upper eyelid. If this is not available, skin from the retroauricular region can be used. Other possible skin donor sites include the supraclavicular skin, the inner arm, and the groin [3].

Prophylactic intubation of the nasolacrimal system with silicone tubes prior to irradiation may help to maintain patency of the nasolacrimal drainage system [2].

Fig. 5. Mechanical basis for ectropion (left) and entropion (right) with appropriate surgical correction through placement of a spacer externally for ectropion repair and internally for entropion repair.

Fig. 6. Radiation-associated conjunctival telangiectasis may persist following the treatment course. The major effect of this is cosmetic, with patients complaining of persistently red eyes.

Conjunctiva, Sclera, and Cornea

Following irradiation of the globe, the conjunctiva may become acutely and transiently injected [4, 5]. Chronic changes include the development of conjunctival telangiectasis, squamous metaplasia, and damage to the accessory lacrimal glands [6, 7] (fig. 6).

Transient keratitis may develop following irradiation. Corneal injury may be complicated by epithelial damage leading to persistent erosions and bacterial infection, and ultimately either corneal scarring or thinning with resultant perforation [8]. The sclera may also become thinned, compromising the integrity of the globe [9–11].

Clinical Syndromes

Conjunctival injection following irradiation is commonly seen and is usually self-limited. Squamous metaplasia of the conjunctiva results in thickening and keratinization of the involved region. Keratinization of the middle portion of the upper eyelid can lead to chronic abrasion of the cornea and recurrent epithelial defects [1] (fig. 7). This potential problem underscores the importance of performing a complete exam with eversion of eyelids before deciding that a recurrent corneal erosion is caused by primary corneal injury. In addition to lid malposition, cicatricial changes of the conjunctiva can cause foreshortening and eventual obliteration of the fornices. This complication is seen most commonly in patients who have undergone enucleation, in some instances compromising their ability to wear a prosthetic [12].

Radiation exposure can lead to primary corneal injury as well. Patients may present with photophobia, ocular discomfort or pain, and some degree of visual loss. Keratitis may be transient or may progress to persistent corneal erosions, scarring, neovascularization, thinning, and perforation [8] (fig. 8). As mentioned previously, manifestations of primary corneal injury may be indistinguishable from those caused by radiation-induced changes to adjacent structures which are necessary for the maintenance of corneal integrity.

Radiation of the sclera can produce thinning, or scleromalacia, of various degrees. Scleral perforation and endophthalmitis following β-irradiation have been described in several cases [9–11, 13] (fig. 9).

Treatment

Squamous metaplasia causing corneal injury is treated with debridement of the abnormal conjunctival tissue and placement of a mucosal graft, often obtained from the buccal surface of the mouth (fig. 10). Following placement of the graft, the lids are sutured together for 1 week to lessen the effects of graft shrinkage [3].

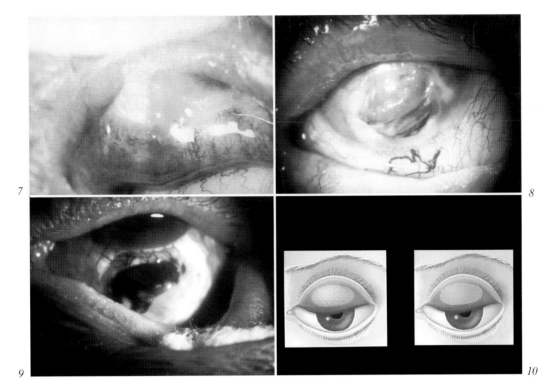

Fig. 7. Scarring and cicatrix on the internal aspect of the upper lid overlying the tarsus following radiation for basal cell carcinoma.

Fig. 8. Corneal perforation with extrusion of the lens following radiation therapy. Corneal perforation can occur for a variety of reasons: Chronic lid changes may result in corneal exposure; dysfunction of the lacrimal apparatus may result in a failure of the tear film's protective function; secondary bacterial infection may result in corneal ulceration and necrosis.

Fig. 9. Radiation-associated scleral necrosis results here in herniation of uveal tissue. This complication is infrequently seen following brachytherapy when the maximum dose to the sclera is appropriately planned. Patients with underlying collagen vascular disease, such as rheumatoid arthritis, may occasionally demonstrate scleral 'melting' following radiation therapy. This complication has also been described in patients receiving β-irradiation.

Fig. 10. Radiation may result in metaplastic conjunctiva with resulting abrasion of the cornea. A conjunctival patch graft can remedy this problem, as shown.

A contracted fornix is managed surgically when a patient is unable to retain a prosthetic globe. One approach to this problem consists of making an incision in the region of the proposed new fornix. Sharp dissection is carried out, and a bed is created for a graft. The graft, obtained from the buccal mucosa, is held in place with interrupted sutures. The conformer is placed in the socket. The lids are then temporarily sutured together, and a tight pressure patch is placed over the eyelids [3].

Treatment of mild conjunctivitis and keratitis is aimed at improving patient comfort and preventing further drying of the globe. Ocular lubricants in either solution or ointment form may be employed. Topical steroids should be used judiciously only in symptomatic patients who are unresponsive to ocular lubricants. Steroids should be withheld in any patient with a confluent epithelial corneal defect since steroids retard re-epithelialization of the cornea and facilitate infection. If a confluent corneal epithelial defect is present, topical antibiotics should be used to prevent bacterial infection. The conjunctiva and tear-producing glands should be evaluated for pathology that may contribute to corneal injury. Dry eye should be treated as well. If steroids are employed chronically, the patient should be followed by an ophthalmologist; a subset of patients will develop steroid-associated glaucoma.

Mild corneal or scleral thinning can be observed; however, severe thinning creates a significant risk of globe perforation. In these cases, surgical management with a patch graft may be warranted. Corneal or scleral tissue may be obtained from donor eyes (fig. 11).

Lacrimal and Accessory Lacrimal Glands

The tear film is comprised of three layers. The conjunctival goblet cells produce the mucous layer which adheres to the hydrophobic corneal surface, giving it hydrophilic properties. The aqueous layer then covers the mucous. The aqueous tear film is produced by both the lacrimal gland and the accessory lacrimal gland tissue within the conjunctiva. The oily layer, produced by the meibomian glands, is spread over the aqueous to prevent evaporation of the underlying layer.

Radiation has been shown to cause damage to a variety of tissues which are responsible for tear production [6, 7]. Damage to any one of these tissues may result in tear film abnormalities and a resultant dry eye (fig. 12). Symptoms of dry eye can be exacerbated by radiation-induced eyelid abnormalities that cause exposure of the cornea or an incomplete blink response.

Clinical Syndromes
Patients with dry eye complain of a sandy-gritty feeling, reflex tearing, burning, or a foreign body sensation. These symptoms usually worsen as the day progresses. As the cornea becomes more involved, the patient may suffer photophobia and increased discomfort.

Rose Bengal and fluorescein stains placed in the tear film are useful in evaluating dry eye. Rose Bengal stains regions of devitalized epithelium and

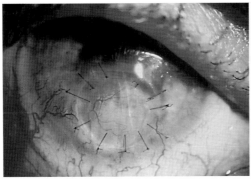
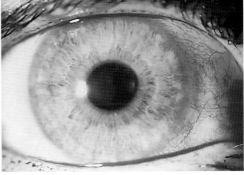

Fig. 11. In cases where corneal perforation has occurred or is imminent, a corneoscleral patch graft (shown here) may be effective.

Fig. 12. Mild cases of dry eye can be diagnosed with Rose Bengal stain, and appropriate treatment with lubricating solutions can obviate future complications.

may detect dry conjunctiva as well as cornea. Fluorescein adheres to basement membrane and will stain regions devoid of epithelial cells. Patients with dry eye will often exhibit a punctate keratopathy, especially of the inferior one-third of the cornea.

Treatment

Mild to moderate symptoms of dry eye can be managed with ocular lubrication. Preservative-free lubricants and the more viscous methylcellulose solutions may be used in more protracted cases. Ointments may be added as well, but because they blur vision, these preparations are better tolerated when used at night. Occasionally, overuse of ocular lubricants with exposure to the various preservatives in the lubricants can exacerbate keratitis. If this is suspected, all drops should be discontinued, and the patient should be observed for improvement. Humidifiers and moist chamber spectacles can be useful, since increasing environmental humidity and retarding evaporation can decrease tear osmolarity.

In severe cases of dry eye, drainage of available tears can be decreased by occluding the puncta. The increased tear volume which results decreases tear film osmolarity. Tear evaporation then has a less drying effect, and freshly secreted tears have an enhanced dilutional effect. Silicone punctal plugs may be used for reversible occlusion of the punctum in order to test patient response to the change in tear volume. These plugs have a dome-shaped top which sits on the surface of the lid, a shaft positioned in the canaliculus, and a wider distal portion which secures the plug in place [14].

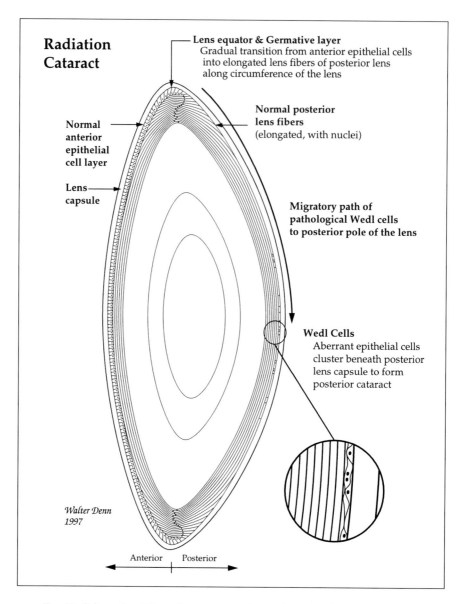

Radiation Cataract

Lens equator & Germative layer
Gradual transition from anterior epithelial cells into elongated lens fibers of posterior lens along circumference of the lens

Normal anterior epithelial cell layer

Lens capsule

Normal posterior lens fibers
(elongated, with nuclei)

Migratory path of pathological Wedl cells to posterior pole of the lens

Wedl Cells
Aberrant epithelial cells cluster beneath posterior lens capsule to form posterior cataract

Walter Denn 1997

Anterior   Posterior

Fig. 13. Schematic of lens showing normal anterior migration as well as aberrant posterior migration of epithelial cells. The abnormal posterior cells, or Wedl cells, cluster along the posterior capsule of the lens forming the posterior subcapsular cataract typically seen following radiation exposure.

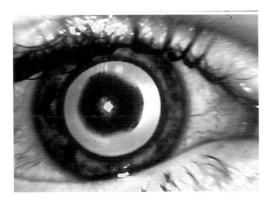

Fig. 14. Posterior subcapsular cataract is frequently seen following radiation therapy and may be visually disabling. Cataract extraction is curative.

Irreversible punctal occlusion is accomplished through scarring of the puncta. In these cases, a low temperature cautery device is inserted into the canaliculus and activated for 1.5–2 s. The inferior puncta is usually closed first. If symptoms persist, the superior puncta may be closed within 8 weeks to months after the initial procedure [14].

Severe cases of corneal drying require further treatment, especially in the setting of a persistent corneal defect. In such instances, the outer portion of the eyelid may be surgically closed to decrease the area of exposed corneal surface.

Lens

Radiation-induced cataracts follow injury to the DNA of the lens epithelial cells which are located in the germinative zone [15, 16]. Wedl cells, or abnormal epithelial cells, migrate to form posterior subcapsular opacities (fig. 13). Ion pump abnormalities have also been implicated in postirradiation cataracts [17–19]. Intraocular tumors, steroid use and intraocular inflammation are all cataractogenic and should be excluded before the lenticular changes are all attributed to radiation damage.

Clinical Syndromes

Following low-dose exposure, the onset of radiation-induced lenticular changes may be delayed. Lens change usually present as a posterior subcapsular opacification (fig. 14); however, anterior subcapsular opacification may precede this [16]. Because these opacities are centrally located, patients are most symptomatic in bright light when the pupils are constricted. Vision may be stable for years, then deteriorate as the cataract matures. Opacification of the lens may also compromise the physician's view into the eye. Such cataracts often create difficulties in ophthalmologic evaluation of intraocular malignancies or other vision-threatening processes which are not optimally visualized through lens opacities.

Treatment

The decision to perform cataract surgery relies primarily on the severity of the patient's symptomatology, as well as the physician's need to view the inside of the eye. The ophthalmologist needs to consider that the visual benefit of cataract surgery for the patient may be compromised by radiation-associated retinopathy or the underlying pathology (e.g. a tumor located in the macula). A potential acuity meter may be used to project the eye chart past the cataract and onto the retina in order to assess the patient's visual potential. Any patient with suspected tumor activity should not undergo cataract extraction due to a potential for tumor dissemination.

Retina

Radiation retinopathy is produced by an occlusive microangiopathy [20–25]. Early changes include focal loss of capillary endothelial cells and pericytes. Regions of acellular capillaries become progressively more confluent leading to microinfarcts seen clinically as cotton-wool spots. These regions may enlarge over time and can be demonstrated on fluorescein angiography as areas of capillary nonperfusion [26]. Vascular injury may result in multifocal regions of inner retinal atrophy, with loss of the ganglion cell layer, and thinning of the nerve fiber layer [27]. Progressive vascular changes may result in microaneurysms and large, dilated vessels with thick collagenous walls. Histologic findings include thickened arteriolar capillary walls, myointimal proliferation, swelling of the endothelium, an enlarged elastic lamina, and narrowing and occlusion of the vessel lumens [28]. Direct damage to photoreceptors and the retinal pigment epithelium has also been reported [29].

Clinical Syndromes

The vascular abnormalities seen in radiation retinopathy cause ischemia of the nerve fiber layer with resultant backup of axoplasmic flow. This is seen clinically as superficial white retinal patches named cotton-wool spots. Microaneurysms and telangiectasis, hemorrhages, macular edema, and intra-

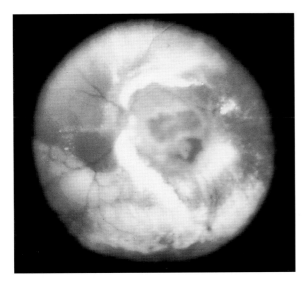

Fig. 15. Wide-angle fundus photo of massive exudative retinopathy following ^{125}I brachy-therapy for the treatment of a choroidal melanoma within the macula.

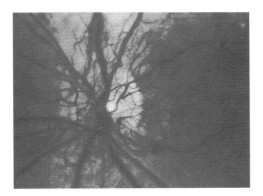

Fig. 16. Neovascularization of the disc can occur in response to ischemic changes in the retina following radiation therapy.

retinal exudates may also be seen [20–25, 30] (fig. 15). Fluorescein angiography usually demonstrates incomplete capillary perfusion of the capillary bed in these areas [20–24, 30, 31]. As in diabetes, radiation-induced retinal ischemia seems to be associated with the formation of neovascular blood vessels (fig. 16). These new abnormal blood vessels may spontaneously bleed, resulting in vitreous hemorrhage or, if associated with fibrous tissue, neovascu-

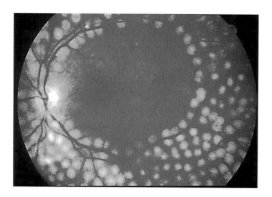

Fig. 17. In the presence of neovascularization, panretinal photocoagulation applied as demonstrated can produce regression of the abnormal vessels and thereby prevent complications such as vitreous hemorrhage or tractional retinal detachment.

lar bands may pull on the retina and cause it to tear or to tractionally detach.

Patients' visual symptoms depend on the part of the retina which is involved. Retinal edema involving the macula can produce loss of central vision. Hemorrhage into the vitreous can result in multiple floaters and decreased visual acuity. On the other hand, peripheral retinal changes often go unnoticed by the patient.

Treatment

Management is aimed at preventing or minimizing visual loss. No clear recommendations exist for treatment of radiation-induced retinopathy; however, because the clinical course of this condition seems to parallel that of diabetic retinopathy, some of the same management principles are often applied.

Laser ablation of incompetent vessels is sometimes used to treat macular edema. Despite treatment, intraretinal fluid may take months to resolve. Since fluid and exudates may be toxic to the photoreceptors, significant recovery of vision is not the rule. Rather, the goal of treatment is to prevent further visual loss.

As in diabetic retinopathy, it is felt that the ischemic retina acts as a stimulus for the development of proliferative neovascular tissue. For this reason, photocoagulation is aimed at ablation of the majority of the peripheral retina (fig. 17). Regression of neovascular tissue following panretinal photocoagulation for radiation retinopathy has been reported [20, 21, 32, 33].

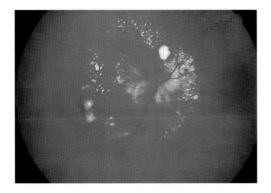

Fig. 18. Following radiation, exudative papillopathy can be seen as in this case, where numerous yellow hard and soft exudates are seen surrounding the disc.

Optic Nerve

As in radiation retinopathy, vascular injury appears to play an important part in the pathogenesis of radiation-induced optic neuropathy [34–36]. Histologic sections show endothelial hyperplasia with narrowing of vessel lumens, fibrinoid necrosis, astrocytic proliferation and demyelination [36].

Clinical Syndromes

Radiation-associated optic neuropathy presents as a sudden, painless, monocular loss of vision [35–39]. Visual loss occurs in a period of days to weeks, and patients may report transient episodes of visual blurring. The appearance of the nerve depends on the portion receiving high-dose radiation. The optic disc may appear normal or be slightly pale following irradiation to the posterior orbit or chiasm [36, 38, 39]. In contrast, the optic nerve head may appear edematous with enlarged tortuous vessels, peripapillary hemorrhages, exudates, cotton-wool spots, and subretinal fluid following irradiation to the eye or anterior optic nerve [35] (fig. 18). Within weeks to months, the edema and hemorrhages subside and are replaced by pallor [36]. Fluorescein angiography demonstrates ischemia of the optic nerve head with areas of capillary nonperfusion and areas of leakage [35].

Treatment

At present, no proven therapy exists for radiation-induced injury to the optic nerve. Initial encouraging results following use of hyperbaric oxygen for treatment of radiation optic neuropathy have not been substantiated by the literature [34, 37].

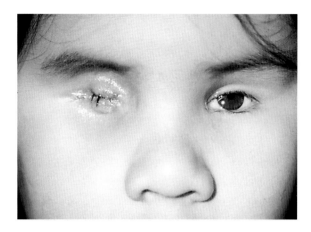

Fig. 19. In this patient, the left socket has undergone oculoplastic reconstruction for cicatricial changes which occurred through poorly fractionated radiation (treatment delivered outside the United States). Reconstruction on the right side has not yet commenced. The patient is wearing an ocular prosthesis on the left and has not yet had an ocular prosthesis placed on the right. Repair required placement of a buccal mucosal membrane graft.

Orbit

Radiation delivered to the orbits of children may arrest bony growth and lead to hypoplasia. The degree of underdevelopment is inversely related to the patient's age during the time of treatment. In addition, orbital soft tissue atrophy may decrease orbital volume and result in posterior displacement of the globe or the prosthetic (fig. 19).

Clinical Syndromes

The effects of external beam irradiation in children treated for retinoblastoma and rhabdomyosarcoma have been well documented [12, 40–42]. The midsection of the face and involved orbit are often hypoplastic in affected patients. Underdevelopment of the nasal bridge, zygomatic bone and temporal fossa, as well as decreased vertical and horizontal orbital diameters, are often demonstrated. The frontal bone may grow normally and can appear disproportionately prominent.

Radiation-induced soft tissue atrophy may result in enophthalmos [12, 40, 41, 43, 44]. This effect is accentuated in the case of an anophthalmic socket, where some degree of volume loss and redistribution of orbital fat may produce downward and posterior displacement of the prosthetic [12]. In unilateral cases, patients may complain of cosmetically unacceptable facial asymmetry.

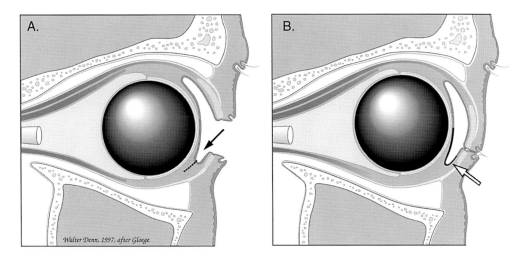

Fig. 20. A Schematic showing foreshortening of the inferior fornix following enucleation and radiation exposure. Note the spherical implant behind the conjunctival surface. The small space inferiorly between the implant and eyelids may compromise fitting of an ocular prosthetic. The dotted line shows where an incision may be made to begin reconstruction of the fornix. *B* Restoration of the inferior fornix following incision with placement of a mucous membrane graft.

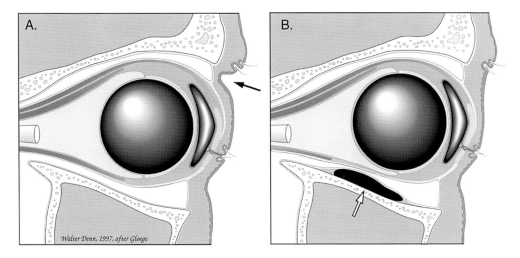

Fig. 21. A Schematic demonstrating enophthalmos following enucleation and radiation. Note posterior displacement of the spherical orbital implant and overlying ocular prosthetic. The superior lid crease may appear deep in these patients (arrow) giving an overall sunken appearance to the prosthetic eye. *B* Placement of an implant in the subperiosteal space in the inferior posterior orbit (arrow) causes upward and anterior movement of the orbital contents and filling out of the upper lid crease.

Heritable retinoblastoma is caused by a germline mutation of the retino-blastoma tumor suppressor gene [45]. Affected children demonstrate an increased incidence of second primary neoplasms throughout their lifetimes. Treatment of retinoblastoma with external beam irradiation increases that risk in children with heritable disease [46–50]. The most common tumor occurring in the field of radiation is osteosarcoma of the orbit, maxilla and nasal bones. Other neoplasms reported include soft tissue sarcomas, leukemia, brain tumors, and melanoma.

Treatment

Enophthalmos occurring in the anophthalmic socket is first managed by fitting a larger prosthetic to compensate for the loss of orbital volume. The weight of the larger prosthetic, however, may produce further downward and posterior displacement of the orbital contents, eventually obviating its own effect. When a cosmetically acceptable result can no longer be achieved, orbital volume augmentation can be performed surgically. One commonly used approach to this problem consists of placing an additional subperiosteal implant in the orbital floor to elevate the orbital contents, which then raises the prosthetic. The lower eyelid can also be surgically tightened to help support the prosthetic [3] (fig. 20, 21).

Acknowledgment

We are very grateful for the expert editorial advice of Sharon Wheeler.

References

1   Fitzpatrick PJ, Thompson GA, Easterbrook WM, Gallie BL, Payne DG: Basal and squamous cell carcinoma of the eyelids and their treatment by radiotherapy. Int J Radiat Oncol Biol Phys 1984; 10:449–454.
2   Lovato AA, Char DH, Castro JR, Kroll SM: The effect of silicone nasolacrimal intubation on epiphora after helium ion irradiation of uveal melanomas. Am J Ophthalmol 1989;108:431–434.
3   McCord CD Jr (ed): Oculoplastic Surgery. New York, Raven Press, 1981.
4   Jereb B, Lee H, Jakobiec FA, Kutcher J: Radiation therapy of conjunctival and orbital lymphoid tumors. Int J Radiat Oncol Biol Phys 1984;10:1013–1019.
5   Dunbar SF, Linggood RM, Doppke KP, Duby A, Wang CC: Conjunctival lymphoma: Results and treatment with a single anterior electron field. A lens sparing approach. Int J Radiat Oncol Biol Phys 1990;19:249–257.
6   Stephens LC, Schultheiss TE, Peters LJ, Ang KK, Gray KN: Acute radiation injury of oclar adnexa. Arch Ophthalmol 1988;106:389–391.
7   Karp LA, Streeten BW, Cogan DG: Radiation-induced atrophy of the meibomian glands. Arch Ophthalmol 1979;97:303–305.
8   Bahrassa F, Datta R: Postoperative beta-radiation treatment of pterygium. Int J Radiat Oncol Biol Phys 1983;9:679–684.

9   MacKenzie FD, Hirst LW, Kynaston B, Bain C: Recurrence rate and complications after beta-irradiation for pterygia. Ophthalmology 1991;98:1776–1780.

10   Tarr KH, Constable IJ: Pseudomonas endophthalmitis associated with scleral necrosis. Br J Ophthalmol 1980;64:676–679.

11   Tarr KH, Constable IJ: Late complications of pterygium treatment. Br J Ophthalmol 1980;64:496–505.

12   Messmer EP, Fritze H, Mohr C, Heinrich T, Sauerwein W, Havers W, Horsthemke B, Hopping W: Long-term treatment effects in patients with bilateral retinoblastoma: Ocular and mid-facial findings. Graefes Arch Clin Exp Ophthalmol 1991;229:309–314.

13   Talbot AN: Complications of beta-ray treatment of pterygia. Trans Ophthalmol Soc NZ 1979;31:62–63.

14   Gilbard JP: Dry eye disorders; in Albert DM, Jakobiec FA (eds): Principles and Practice of Ophthalmology. Philadelphia, Saunders, 1994, vol 1, pp 257–276.

15   Worgul BV, Merriam GR, Szechter A, Srinivasan D: Lens epithelium and radiation cataract: Preliminary studies. Arch Ophthalmol 1976;94:996–999.

16   Cogan DG, Donaldson DD, Reese AB: Clinical and pathological characteristics of radiation cataract. Arch Ophthalmol 1952;47:55–70.

17   Matsuda H, Giblin FJ, Reddy VN: The effect of X-irradiation on the Na-K-ATPase and cation distribution in rabbit lens. Invest Ophthalmol Vis Sci 1982;22:180–185.

18   Hightower KR, Giblin FJ, Reddy VN: Changes in the distribution of lens calcium during development of X-ray cataract. Invest Ophthalmol Vis Sci 1983;24:1188–1193.

19   Lambert BW, Kinoshita JH: The effects of ionizing irradiation on lens cation permeability, transport, and hydration. Invest Ophthalmol Vis Sci 1967;6:624–634.

20   Thompson GM, Migdal CS, Whittle RJ: Radiation retinopathy following treatment of posterior nasal space carcinoma. Br J Ophthalmol 1983;67:609–614.

21   Lopez PF, Sternberg P Jr, Dabbs CK, Vogler WR, Crocker I, Kalin NS: Bone marrow transplant retinopathy. Am J Ophthalmol 1991;112:635–646 (Erratum: Am J Ophthalmol 1992;113:616).

22   Brown GC, Shields JA, Sanborn G, Augsburger JJ, Savino PJ, Schatz NJ: Radiation retinopathy. Ophthalmology 1982;89:1494–1501.

23   Noble KG, Kupersmith MJ: Retinal vascular remodelling in radiation retinopathy. Br J Ophthalmol 1984;68:475–478.

24   Hayreh SS: Post-radiation retinopathy. A fluorescence fundus angiographic study. Br J Ophthalmol 1970;54:705–714.

25   Gass JD: A fluorescein angiographic study of macular dysfunction secondary to retinal vascular disease. X-ray irradiation, carotid artery occlusion, collagen vascular disease, and vitritis. Arch Ophthalmol 1968;80:606–617.

26   Irvine AR, Wood IS: Radiation retinopathy as an experimental model for ischemic proliferative retinopathy and rubeosis iridis. Am J Ophthalmol 1987;103:790–797.

27   Boozalis GT, Schachat AP, Green WR: Subretinal neovascularization from the retina in radiation retinopathy. Retina 1987;7:156–161.

28   Egbert PR, Fajardo LF, Donaldson SS, Moazed K: Posterior ocular abnormalities after irradiation for retinoblastoma: A histopathological study. Br J Ophthalmol 1980;64:660–665.

29   Amoaku WM, Frew L, Mahon GJ, Gardiner TA, Archer DB: Early ultrastructural changes after low-dose X-irradiation in the retina of the rat. Eye 1989;3:638–646.

30   Wara WM, Irvine AR, Neger RE, Howes EL Jr, Phillips TL: Radiation retinopathy. Int J Radiat Oncol Biol Phys 1979;5:81–83.

31   Midena E, Segato T, Piermarocchi S, Corti L, Zorat PL, Moro F: Retinopathy following radiation therapy of paranasal sinus and nasopharyngeal carcinoma. Retina 1987;7:142–147.

32   Chaudhuri PR, Austin DJ, Rosenthal AR: Treatment of radiation retinopathy. Br J Ophthalmol 1981;65:623–625.

33   Kinyoun JL, Chittum ME, Wells CG: Photocoagulation treatment of radiation retinopathy. Am J Ophthalmol 1988;105:470–478.

34   Guy J, Schatz NJ: Hyperbaric oxygen in the treatment of radiation-induced optic neuropathy. Ophthalmology 1986;93:1083–1088.

35 Brown GC, Shields JA, Sanborn G, Augsburger JJ, Savino PJ, Schatz NJ: Radiation optic neuropathy. Ophthalmology 1982;89:1489–1493.
36 Kline LB, Kim JY, Ceballos R: Radiation optic neuropathy. Ophthalmology 1985;92:1118–1126.
37 Roden D, Bosley TM, Fowble B, Clark J, Savino PJ, Sergott RC, Schatz NJ: Delayed radiation injury to the retrobulbar optic nerves and chiasm. Clinical syndrome and treatment with hyperbaric oxygen and corticosteroids. Ophthalmology 1990;97:346–351.
38 Zimmerman CF, Schatz NJ, Glaser JS: Magnetic resonance imaging of radiation optic neuropathy. Am J Ophthalmol 1990;110:389–394.
39 Guy J, Mancuso A, Quisling RG, Beck R, Moster M: Gadolinium-DTPA-enhanced magnetic resonance imaging in optic neuropathies. Ophthalmology 1990;97:592–600.
40 Heyn R, Ragab A, Raney RB Jr, Ruymann F, Tefft M, Lawrence W Jr, Soule E, Maurer HM: Late effects of therapy in orbital rhabdomyosarcoma in children. A report from the Intergroup Rhabdomyosarcoma Study. Cancer 1986;57:1738–1743.
41 Larson DL, Kroll S, Jaffe N, Serure A, Goepfert H: Long-term effects of radiotherapy in childhood and adolescence. Am J Surg 1990;160:348–351.
42 Malbran J: Facial changes due to radiation in cases of retinoblastoma. Ophthalmologica 1969;157:268–273.
43 Fiorillo A, Migliorati R, Grimaldi M, Vassallo P, Canale G, Tranfa F, Uccello G, Fiore M, Muto P, Menna G, Parasole R, Bonavolonta G: Multidisciplinary treatment of primary orbital rhabdomyosarcoma: A single-institution experience. Cancer 1991;67:560–563.
44 Haik BG, Jereb B, Smith ME, Ellsworth RM, McCormick B: Radiation and chemotherapy of parameningeal rhabdomyosarcoma involving the orbit. Ophthalmology 11986;93:1001–1009.
45 Friend SH, Bernards R, Rogelj S, Weinberg RA, Rapaport JM, Albert DM, Dryja TP: A human DNA segment with properties of the gene that predisposes to retinoblastoma and osteosarcoma. Nature 1986;323:643–646.
46 Abramson DH, Ellsworth RM, Kitchin FD, Tung G: Second nonocular tumors in retinoblastoma survivors: Are they radiation-induced? Ophthalmology 1984;91:1351–1355.
47 Roarty JD, McLean IW, Zimmerman LE: Incidence of second neoplasms in patients with bilateral retinoblastoma. Ophthalmology 1988;95:1583–1587.
48 Draper GJ, Sanders BM, Kingston JE: Second primary neoplasms in patients with retinoblastoma. Br J Cancer 1986;53:661–671.
49 Tucker MA, D'Angio GJ, Boice JD Jr, Strong LC, Li FP, Stovall M, Stone BJ, Green DM, Lombardi F, Newton W, Hoover RN, Fraumeni JF Jr: Bone sarcomas linked to radiotherapy and chemotherapy in children. N Engl J Med 1987;317:588–593.
50 Schwarz MB, Burgess LP, Fee WE Jr, Donaldson SS: Postirradiation sarcoma in retinoblastoma. Induction or predisposition? Arch Otolaryngol Head Neck Surg 1988;114:640–644.

Kathleen B. Gordon, MD, Department of Ophthalmology, University of California, San Francisco, 10 Kirkham Street, Box 0730, San Francisco, CA 94143-0730 (USA)

Meyer JL (ed): Radiation Injury. Advances in Management and Prevention.
Front Radiat Ther Oncol. Basel, Karger, 1999, vol 32, pp 145–154

....

Radiation Injury to the Central Nervous System: Clinical Features and Prevention

K. Kian Ang

Department of Radiation Oncology, UTMD Anderson Cancer Center,
Houston, Tex., USA

Introduction

Chronic iatrogenic neurotoxicity manifests in three clinical entities depending on the site and volume of the central nervous system (CNS) affected. Briefly, injury to the spinal cord and brainstem results in neurologic (sensory and/or motor) deficits which can lead to lethality. Damage to the cerebrum produces neurologic deficit, cognitive impairment, or both depending on the radiation portal, volume, and dose. Injury to the hypothalamus-pituitary system induces neuroendocrine anomaly.

CNS injury is generally ranked as one of the most serious complications because it decreases the quality of life of affected patients and no effective treatment is available with the exception of hormonal substitution for some of the neuroendocrine dysfunctions. Therefore, radiation oncologists often limit the dose to the CNS to well below the threshold level of radiation injury to avoid the occurrence of this dramatic complication. Because of the central location, the tolerance of the spinal cord to radiation is considered a major dose-limiting factor and hence an obstacle to curing some neoplasms located in or around the neuraxis by radiotherapy.

A consequence of the conservative approach of keeping the radiation dose well below the threshold level, sometimes at the cost of underdosage of the tumor, is that clinical material on radiation-induced spinal cord injury (myelopathy) is scarce. As a result, clinical practice has been dominated by dogmas and assumptions. Numerous animal studies have been undertaken during the last two decades to address some of the prevailing dogmas, elucidate the pathology-pathogenesis of CNS injury, and to identify determinants of CNS tolerance. A large body of clinically applicable data has been generated. The objective of this chapter is to summarize the clinical features and available human data on iatrogenic neurotoxicity and to present a few guidelines for prevention of CNS toxicity developed from results of experimental studies. The primary focus is to review the treatment-induced late neurologic deficits.

Clinical Features of Iatrogenic Neurotoxicity

Cognitive Impairment

Iatrogenic intellectual dysfunction occurs gradually after therapy. It is detected by a battery of cognitive tests such as Wechsler Intelligence Scale for Children-Revised (WISC-R, which measures full-scale, verbal and performance IQs), Wide Range Achievement Test (WRAT, which evaluates reading, spelling, and arithmetic abilities), etc. A confounding factor in quantifying the magnitude of decline in intelligence is the existence of a wide spectrum of interindividual variations in the general population.

Cognitive impairments have been more extensively documented in children who were cured of acute lymphoblastic leukemia (ALL). The vast majority of these children received a combination of cranial irradiation (CI) and intrathecal methotrexate (ITMTX) or triple intrathecal chemotherapy (MTX, ara-C, and hydrocortisone) as elective treatment to the CNS. A consistent finding from retrospective studies is that children who received 24 Gy CI and ITMTX or triple intrathecal chemotherapy scored slightly but steadily lower (by ~10 points) on full-scale IQ, performance IQ, arithmetic, etc., than the controls [1, 2]. However, children who received 18 Gy CI plus ITMTX performed at the same level as controls [2]. These data reveal that the threshold dose of CI (administered with ITMTX) for inducing a mild, diffuse information processing deficit is between 18 Gy in 10 fractions and 24 Gy in 12 fractions.

There is evidence that younger children tend to develop more severe neuropsychological dysfunction after CI and ITMTX therapy [3, 4]. In Halberg's series [2], 8 of 9 children with IQ scores of <90 had received CI before age 5. This observation provided the impetus for developing high-dose chemotherapy CNS prophylaxis. A prospective trial was designed to address the relative toxicity of *parenteral methotrexate* versus CI [5]. In this study, children who achieved complete remission with induction chemotherapy were randomized to receive either cranial irradiation (RT group) or intravenous methotrexate (MTX group) as CNS prophylaxis. Children in the RT group received 18 Gy CI in 12 fractions plus 5 concurrent doses of ITMTX; those in the MTX group received a total of 15 intravenous infusions of 1 g/m^2 methotrexate (first 3 at weekly interval then every 6 weeks) and ITMTX.

Patients were tested immediately after remission induction, then at yearly intervals until the cessation of therapy, and subsequently every other year over the next 5 years. The test results show that mean scores for intelligence or academic achievements did not differ between the two groups. With the exception of final arithmetic scores, means for tests of intelligence or academic achievements were not significantly different from those for a normative population. However, statistically significant decreases in full-scale IQ, verbal IQ, and arithmetic achievement were found within both groups. Clinically important decreases (≥ 15 points) on one or more neuropsychological measures occurred in 14 of 23 patients in the RT group and in 16 of 26 children in the MTX group. General follow-up evaluations revealed that 15 patients in the RT group had somnolence syndrome and 4 developed cerebral calcifications late in their clinical course. In the MTX group, 15 had abnormal electroencephalograms and 6 had early, transient white-matter hypodensities on computerized tomogram (CT) scans. There were no correlations between these changes and the neuropsychological test results. It was concluded that 18 Gy CI and parenteral methotrexate are associated with comparable decreases in neuropsychologic functions. The lack of a deficit pattern suggests, however, that other factors such as school absences and delayed development due to illness may have contributed to decreased cognitive functions.

Radiation-Induced Late Neurologic Deficit
Clinical Presentation
Focal cerebral necrosis is the typical late effect of therapeutic or incidental brain irradiation. The onset is generally between 6 months and 2 years after therapy. Symptoms and signs include site-specific focal deficits (e.g. paresis, paresthesia, aphasia, etc.), seizures, and symptoms of intracranial hypertension. CT scans usually reveal low-density white-matter changes with irregular enhancement often associated with surrounding diffuse edema and a variable degree of mass effect confined to the high-dose volume. MRI shows similar changes and often identifies more pronounced white-matter edema [6]. Differentiation from tumor recurrence or progression may be difficult.

Focal brain necrosis has rarely been observed at doses < 60 Gy for conventionally fractionated external beam irradiation [7, 8]. A threshold of 57.6 Gy has been reported for daily irradiation with fraction sizes < 2 Gy [9]. The incidence is highly dependent upon fraction size. Most reported necroses following 'incidental' brain irradiation have occurred with fractions of > 2.2–2.5 Gy [8].

In patients with brain neoplasms, it is important to recognize the *subacute encephalopathy* syndrome. This syndrome manifests most frequently 2–6 months after therapy as fatigue, somnolence, and exacerbation of focal neurologic symptoms and signs. It may be difficult to differentiate this usually transient syndrome from tumor progression, which might even lead to the prescription of additional therapy for presumed disease recurrence [6].

Radiation myelopathy can have a subtle onset after a latency of usually more than 5–6 months. Objective signs and symptoms include changes in gait (often foot drop), spasticity, weakness, hemiparesis, and less frequently Brown-Sequard syndrome (ipsilateral paralysis and loss of discriminatory sensation and contralateral loss of pain and temperature sensation), incontinence, and occasionally pain. In many cases, the patient may have been asymptomatic until some trauma initiated a progressive neurological deficit.

The dose-incidence relationship is reasonably well established in adults (also see below). A literature review by Schultheiss and Stephens [10] indicates that a total dose of 45 Gy in 22–25 fractions results in $\leq 0.2\%$ incidence of myelopathy. A realistic estimate of the ED_5 (5% complications) for 2-Gy fractions is between 57 and 61 Gy. There is no firm clinical data to support the general belief that the radiation tolerance of the spinal cord in children is much lower than that in adults, as only very few cases of childhood radiation myelopathy have been reported [11]. However, those few cases were observed after doses of about 40 Gy delivered in <2 Gy/fraction. Therefore, it is reasonable to assume a lower tolerance in clinical practice and thus apply approximately a 10% dose reduction in children.

Diagnosis and Pathology

Since no combination of symptoms or signs are specific for radiation-induced focal brain necrosis and myelopathy, the diagnosis of these complications is still made by exclusion. Factors to be taken into account are spatial and temporal relationship with radiation, radiation dose and absence of other causes of CNS injury. The symptom complex may sometimes be helpful in making the differentiation diagnosis. For example, existence of upper extremity symptoms without lower extremity symptoms is a strong argument to eliminate radiation myelopathy as the cause of neurologic deficit. It should also be realized that by far the most common cause for CNS damage in a cancer patient is tumor progression or metastases. The available diagnostic imaging techniques can usually identify tumor progression as the cause of CNS injury. In cases of uncertainty, further follow-up generally resolves the differential diagnosis.

The histopathology of iatrogenic CNS injury has been characterized in human myelopathy cases and evaluated more extensively in rodent and primate myelopathy models [12, 13]. These studies show that radiation myelopathy has no pathognomonic features. The most commonly encountered pathology was prominent white-matter necrosis with minor or no vascular changes. Less frequently, the lesion was composed of a mixture of white-matter necrosis and obvious vasculopathies (combinations of telangiectasis, hyaline degeneration, thrombosis, fibrinoid necrosis, and hemorrhage).

Prevention of Iatrogenic Late Neurologic Deficit

As mentioned earlier, no specific treatment can result in restoration of neurologic function in patients with established radiation-induced CNS necrosis. Treatment with steroids and, in selected cases, surgical resection of the necrotic region can achieve a substantial symptomatic relief by reducing intracranial hypertension in some patients with localized brain necrosis. Therefore, effort should be paid to minimize the risk for inducing CNS injury in various clinical contexts. Obviously, since late effects never have their onset before completion of radiation treatment, there is no opportunity to adjust the dose based on the severity of tissue reactions during radiotherapy. Consequently, therapeutic decisions can be made only on a probability basis based on the available data. It should be kept in mind that in the vast majority of cancers, a reasonable cure rate can only be obtained with radiation doses that are associated with a certain risk of normal tissue damage. What risk is 'acceptable' in a given case depends on a number of factors such as the proximity of the tumor to the CNS, geometry of the lesion, change of tumor control probability with dose increment, etc. A number of useful guidelines to minimize complications are as follows:

Apply Dose-Response Data Rationally
Figure 1 shows the dose-response data for myelopathy obtained in a rhesus monkey model along with relatively large series of reported human myelopathy cases. The estimated doses for 50% (ED_{50}) and 1% myelopathy in rhesus monkey are 76.1 ± 1.9 and 59.1 ± 5.5 Gy, respectively. These values are consistent with the human data, reviewed by Schultheiss et al. [14], revealing that a dose of 45 Gy in 22–25 fractions results in $\leq 0.2\%$ incidence of myelopathy and that a realistic estimate of 5% myelopathy for 2-Gy fractions is 57–61 Gy.

Fortunately, with proper treatment setup and beam orientation, it is possible to deliver desirable therapeutic doses to the tumor (e.g. 70–72 Gy in 35–40 fractions) without exceeding 45 Gy in 22–25 fractions to the spinal cord in most cllinical situations. Based on data presented in figure 1, however, it is reasonable to deliver a dose of 50 Gy in 25 fractions to the spinal cord in an otherwise healthy patient to allow better coverage of disease situated in the proximity of the neuraxis. Such therapy strategy carries an extremely low risk

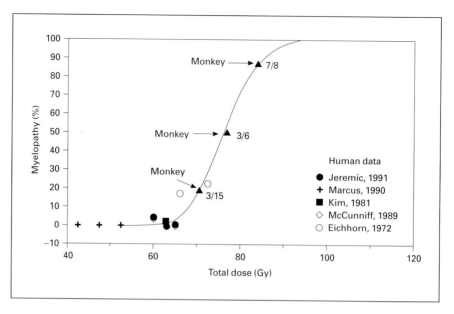

Fig. 1. Dose-incidence relationship for radiation-induced myelopathy in rhesus monkeys receiving irradiation to the cervical spinal cord with 2.2-Gy fractions and reported cases of human myelopathy after irradiation of cervical or thoracic spinal cord with 1.5- to 3.1-Gy fractions.

of inducing myelopathy. On rare occasions, because of the disease extent (e.g. patients with nasopharyngeal carcinoma with involvement of retropharyngeal nodes) good coverage of the tumor volume to therapeutic dose may not be possible without accepting delivery of 50–53 Gy to a small segment of the spinal cord. This therapy plan may be reasonable as the gain in tumor control probability may outweigh the risk of myelopathy. Obviously, it is necessary to inform and involve the patient in treatment decisionmaking when this need arises.

Avoid Short Interaction Intervals

The impact of the interval between irradiations on the rates of CNS toxicity has gained attention because of recent interest in attempting to improve tumor control by altered fractionation regimens. These unconventional regimens require delivery of two or three irradiations a day and thus necessitate shortening of the interfraction intervals from the standard 24 h to 4–6 h. An experimental study on repair kinetics in adult rat spinal cord by Ang et al. [13] showed that cellular repair of sublethal lesions proceeded at a slower rate than previously anticipated. It was found that a biexponential model fit the data better than a monoexponential model. Analysis with a biexponential model revealed a repair half-time ($T_{1/2}$) of 0.7 h for the faster component and a $T_{1/2}$ of 3.8 h for the slower component. As a result, shortening the interfraction interval from 24 h to 8 or 6 h leads to about 10 or 15% reduction in the isoeffective dose, respectively. The higher than expected incidence of myelopathy after 3 fraction/day regimens [15] can at least partly be attributed to compounding incomplete repair between fractions.

Minimize Radiation Treatment Volume

It has been generally accepted that the dose to the spinal cord should be reduced when the volume, i.e. the length of spinal cord, to be irradiated is increased. Clinical data on this subject are, however, scanty and inconclusive. Rodent models have been used to address the effects of irradiating 2-mm to 3-cm segments of spinal cord [16, 17]. It was found that the ED_{50} for white-matter necrosis increases markedly with the reduction of field size from 16 to 4 mm long (21.5 vs. 50.98 Gy for single exposure). However, the increase of ED_{50} for vascular lesions is less pronounced (20 vs. 25.58 Gy). A plausible explanation for this phenomenon is that glial progenitors from unirradiated regions could migrate some distance into the irradiated area. A potential clinical application of these results is in radiosurgery. The data suggest that a thin segment of normal-appearing CNS tissues surrounding metastatic deposits could tolerate a high radiation dose.

Recently, larger animal models (monkey, dog, and pig) were used to evaluate the relationship between radiation volume and cord tolerance for portal sizes used routinely in the clinic. The results in primates and pigs indicate that the influence of the volume on the tolerance dose is consistent with the probability model [18, 19]. The essence of this model is that an increase in the treatment volume reduces the threshold and steepens the slope of the sigmoid dose-response curve for myelopathy. The consequence of the change in the slope of the sigmoid dose-response curve is that the influence of volume on the tolerance dose is less pronounced at low incidence levels (e.g. 1–5% incidence) than at high incidence levels. For example, doubling the treatment volume leads to only an approximately 4% reduction of isoeffect dose at 1–5% incidence level. This means that in treatment settings where the probability of myelopathy is <1%, such as definitive radiotherapy for head and neck and lung cancers, changes in treatment volume have minimal impact on the cord tolerance. However, when a relatively high radiation dose is to be administered, such as in the treatment of brainstem tumors, progressive portal reductions to deliver the highest dose to a small volume (e.g. by 3-D conformal therapy) would reduce the risk for necrosis.

Adjust Radiation Dose to Patient Age

Clinical data suggest that the radiation tolerance of the spinal cord of children may be lower than that of adults, as the few cases of childhood myelopathy were observed after doses of about 40 Gy delivered in <2 Gy/fraction [11]. Ruifrok et al. [20] addressed this issue in rodents. They revealed several interesting findings. Briefly, compared to adult animals, the ED_{50} for 1-week-old rats is ~10% lower (19.5 vs. 21 Gy for single radiation exposure), the latency for myelopathy is substantially shorter (~2 weeks vs. ~8 months), and the fractionation sensitivity is lower or expressed in terms of linear-quadratic (LQ) model for dose response the α/β ratio is higher (4.5 vs. 1.8 Gy). This difference in fractionation sensitivity may lead to a larger difference in the tolerance dose when radiation is fractionated. However, there is evidence that the proliferation kinetics is also faster in immature animals. Proliferation may neutralize the consequence of lower fractionation sensitivity in protracted fractionation regimens. Based on the available clinical and experimental data, it is reasonable to assume a lower tolerance in clinical practice and thus apply approximately 10% dose reduction in the pediatric population.

Beware of Potential Enhancement of Response by Cytotoxic Agents

Chemotherapeutic agents, particularly those that cross the blood-brain barrier and are neurotoxic by themselves, may enhance radiation injury to the CNS. Cytotoxic agents tested and found to modify CNS tolerance in animal models are ara-C, fludarabine, and mitotane [21–24]. Methotrexate administered intrathecally or intraventricularly before irradiation was found to result in a slight radioprotection, i.e. 6–9% increase in the isoeffective doses for white-matter necrosis [21, 25]. In contrast, MTX given during or after irradiation has no detectable modifying effect [25]. These findings are recently supported by clinical data in children with ALL receiving ITMTX and CI in a different sequence [26].

Agents investigated and found to have no modifying effect are: AZQ [27], actinomycin, BCNU, and vincristine [28]. It should be realized that the neurotoxicity of many combined therapy regimens have not been tested in experimental models. In addition, because of potential differences in pharmacokinetics, it may not be prudent to extrapolate quantitative data obtained from experimental studies directly to the clinic.

Summary and Future Directions

The dramatic nature of radiation-induced CNS injury causes clinicians to avoid this complication, sometimes even by compromising tumor control probability. As a result of this practice, clinical material on radiation myelopathy is limited. Radiation biologists have contributed data relevant for clinical practice. Experimental studies have helped in establishing realistic estimates of the dose-incidence relationship, repair parameters, volume and age effects, etc. Concepts and parameters gained from such laboratory studies have been useful for the development of radiotherapy strategies to maximize tumor control probability.

Further advancement in therapeutic strategies, however, must come from elucidation of the pathogenesis of radiation-induced CNS injury since such knowledge is essential for attempting to develop rational approaches for modulating radiation damage to increase the tolerance of the CNS. Recent developments in neurobiology have provided insights into the structural and functional organization of the nervous system. This knowledge is being applied in investigating the pathogenesis of radiation myelopathy and characterizing the temporal progression of radiation-induced lesions.

References

1 Copeland DR, Dowell REJ, Fletcher JM, Bordeaux JD, Sullivan MP, Jaffe N, Frankel LS, Ried HL, Cangir A: Neuropsychological effects of childhood cancer treatment. J Child Neurol 1988;3: 53–62.
2 Halberg FE, Kramer JH, Moore IM, Wara WM, Matthay KK, Ablin AR: Prophylactic cranial irradiation dose effects on late cognitive function in children treated for acute lymphoblastic leukemia. Int J Radiat Oncol Biol Phys 1992;22:13–16.
3 Eiser C, Lansdown R: Retrospective study of intellectual development in children treated for acute lymphoblastic leukemia. Arch Dis Child 1977;52:525–529.
4 Jannoun K: Are cognitive and educational development affected by age at which prophylactic therapy is given in acute lymphoblastic leukemia? Arch Dis Child 1983;58:953–958.
5 Ochs J, Mulhern R, Fairclough D, Parvey L, Whitaker J, Ch'ien L, Mauer A, Simone J: Comparison of neuropsychologic functioning and clinical indicators of neurotoxicity in long-term survivors of childhood leukemia given cranial radiation or parenteral methotrexate: A prospective study. J Clin Oncol 1991;9:145–151.
6 Valk PE, Dillon WP: Diagnostic imaging of central nervous system radiation injury; in Gutin P, Leibel S, Sheline G (eds): Radiation Injury to the Nervous System. New York, Raven Press, 1991, pp 211–237.
7 Kramer S: Radiation effect and tolerance of the central nervous system. Front Radiat Ther Oncol. Basel, Karger, 1972, vol 6, pp 332–345.
8 Sheline GE, Wara WM, Smith V: Therapeutic irradiation and brain injury. Int J Radiat Oncol Biol Phys 1980;6:1215–1228.
9 Leibel SA, Sheline GE: Tolerance of the brain and spinal cord to conventional irradiation; in Gutin P, Leibel SA, Sheline GE (eds): Radiation Injury to the Nervous System. New York, Raven Press, 1991, pp 239–256.
10 Schultheiss TE, Stephens LC: Pathology of radiation myelopathy, widening the circle. Int J Radiat Oncol Biol Phys 1992;23:1089–1091.
11 Sundaresan N, Gutierrez FA, Larsen MB: Radiation myelopathy in children. Ann Neurol 1978;4: 47–50.
12 Schultheiss T, Stephens L, Maor M: Analysis of the histopathology of radiation myelopathy. Int J Radiat Oncol Biol Phys 1988;14:27–32.

13   Ang KK, Price RE, Stephens LC, Jiang GL, Feng Y, Schultheiss TE, Peters LJ: The tolerance of primate spinal cord to re-irradiation. Int J Radiat Oncol Biol Phys 1993;25:459–464.

14   Schultheiss TE, Kun LE, Ang KK, Stephens LC: Radiation response of the central nervous system. Int J Radiat Oncol Biol Phys 1995;31:1093–1112.

15   Dische S: Accelerated treatment and radiation myelitis (editorial). Radiother Oncol 1991;20:1–2.

16   Hopewell JW, Morris AD, Dixon-Brown A: The influence of field size on the late tolerance of the rat spinal cord to single doses of X-rays. Br J Radiol 1987;60:1099–1108.

17   Van der Kogel AJ: Effect of volume and localization on rat spinal cord tolerance; in Fielden EM, Fowler JF, Hendry JH, Scott D (eds): Proc 8th Int Congr Radiation Research. London, Taylor & Francis, 1987, vol 1, p 352.

18   Schultheiss TE, Stephens LC, Ang KK, Price RE, Peters LJ: Volume effects in rhesus monkey spinal cord. Int J Radiat Oncol Biol Phys 1994;29:67–72.

19   Van den Aardweg GJMJ, Hopewell JW, Whitehouse EM: The radiation response of the cervical spinal cord of the pig: Effects of changing the irradiated volume. Int J Radiat Oncol Biol Phys 1995;31:51–55.

20   Ruifrok ACC, Kleiboer BJ, van der Kogel AJ: Radiation tolerance and fractionation sensitivity of the developing rat cervical spinal cord. Int J Radiat Oncol Biol Phys 1992;24:505–510.

21   Van der Kogel AJ, Sissingh HA: Effects of intrathecal methotrexate and cytosine arabinoside on the radiation tolerance of the rat spinal cord. Radiother Oncol 1985;4:239–251.

22   Menten J, Landuyt W, van der Kogel AJ, Ang KK, van der Schueren E: Effects of high-dose intraperitoneal cytosine arabinoside on the radiation tolerance of the rat spinal cord. Int J Radiat Oncol Biol Phys 1989;17:131–134.

23   Gregoire V, Ruifrok ACC, Price RE, Brock WA, Hittelman WN, Plunkett WK, Ang KK: Effect of intraperitoneal fludarabine on rat spinal cord tolerance to fractionated irradiation. Radiother Oncol 1995;36:50–55.

24   Glicksman AS, Bliven SF, Leith JT: Modification of radiation damage in rat spinal cord by mitotane. Cancer Treat Rep 1982;66:1545–1547.

25   Geyer JR, Taylor EM, Milstein JM, Shaw CM, Hubbard BA, Geraci JP, Thornquist M, Bleyer WA: Radiation methotrexate, and white matter necrosis: Laboratory evidence for neural radioprotection with preirradiation methotrexate. Int J Radiat Oncol Biol Phys 1988;15:373–375.

26   Balsom WR, Bleyer WA, Robison LL, Heyn RM, Meadows AT, Sitarz A, Blatt J, Sather HN, Hammond GD: Intellectual function in long-term survivors of childhood acute lymphoblastic leukemia: Protective effect of pre-irradiation methotrexate? A children's cancer study group study. Med Pediatr Oncol 1991;19:486–492.

27   Ang KK, van der Kogel AJ, van der Schueren E: Effect of combined AZQ and radiation on the tolerance of the rat spinal cord. J Neurooncol 1986;3:349–352.

28   Van der Kogel AJ, Scherer E, Streffer C, Trott KR: The nervous system: Radiobiology and experimental pathology; in Scherer E, Streffer C, Trott KR (eds): Medical Radiology. Diagnostic Imaging and Radiation Oncology Radiopathology of Organs and Tissues. Heidelberg, Springer-Verlag, 1991, pp 191–212.

Kian Ang, MD, Division of Radiation Oncology, MD Anderson Cancer Center,
1515 Holcombe Boulevard, Houston, TX 77030 (USA)

Meyer JL (ed): Radiation Injury. Advances in Management and Prevention.
Front Radiat Ther Oncol. Basel, Karger, 1999, vol 32, pp 155–165

....

Management of the Radiosurgery Patient: Causes and Treatment of Adverse Sequelae

Steven D. Chang, John R. Adler

Department of Neurosurgery, Stanford Medical Center, Stanford, Calif., USA

Radiosurgery

The term *radiosurgery* describes several related techniques which combine stereotactic principles of localization with a highly collimated high-energy radiation source. This procedure makes it possible to deliver a very large dose of radiation to a small intracranial lesion while achieving rapid fall-off outside the target volume. Since Leksell [1] pioneered this technique in 1951, it has proven an effective alternative for conventional neurosurgery, cranial irradiation, and brachytherapy in the management of selected small intracranial tumors and arteriovenous malformations (AVMs). Following the rapid proliferation of radiosurgery centers worldwide and the marked increase in the number of patients treated with these methods, the complications of stereotactic radiosurgery are now becoming much better understood.

Adverse sequelae from radiation are broadly classified according to the time of appearance with respect to treatment [2]. Complications from radiosurgery have been similarly categorized. Acute reactions are defined as occurring during, immediately after, or within the first several days of therapy. Early reactions are defined as those that develop within a few weeks to several months after radiosurgery. Late reactions occur more than 3 months following therapy. Acute and early sequelae are generally self-limiting, with no long-term deficits, while late reactions are usually associated with some degree of permanent neurological injury.

Acute Complications

Because of the large fraction size, the potential for acute sequelae is greater with stereotactic radiosurgery than with fractionated radiotherapy. The time course suggests an epigenetic effect of ionizing radiation, with the possible production of free radicals which result in either acute cell death or temporary disruption of the blood-brain barrier [3–5]. Although the exact mechanisms for this phenomenon are poorly understood, acute side effects are short-lived.

Nausea and Emesis

Nausea and emesis are a common acute sequela after radiosurgical treatment of posterior fossa lesions. These symptoms occur in 10–16% of patients within 6 h of treatment [6, 7], and are related to a direct effect on the area postrema [7, 8]. In Loeffler's series [7] of 44 patients, the 7 patients who developed nausea and emesis had a median dose of 618 cGy (range 275–1,257) to the area postrema, compared with the remaining 37 asymptomatic patients who received <500 cGy. These side effects rarely occur beyond 24 h after radiosurgery. Preventive measures include pretreatment with antiemetics and steroids [7, 8]. In our experience at Stanford, newer classes of antiemetics, such as ondansetron, seem to provide virtually complete protection from these symptoms [8].

Acute Neurologic Deterioration from Edema

Acute neurologic deterioration after radiosurgery is unusual. However, in our experience it is more common than published reports would lead us to believe. Loeffler et al. [7] reported 1 patient (1 of 44 – 2%) who developed motor aphasia 1 h following radiosurgical treatment of a recurrent left temporal glioma, which resolved within 12 h. McKenzie et al. [9] reported on 1 patient (1 of 112 – 1%) treated for a left occipital AVM who developed a right homonymous hemianopsia which lasted 8 h. It is logically theorized that such deterioration is caused by acute edema at the treatment site. Glucocorticoids should shorten the duration of symptoms.

Seizures

While seizures and headaches not infrequently occur after stereotactic radiosurgery, these symptoms are also in themselves associated with the underlying pathology in many patients. Consequently it is not always clear when a seizure is directly related to treatment. Kjellberg et al. [10] reported a small increase in acute seizure risk in patients treated with proton radiosurgery. Similarly it has been our experience at Stanford that there is an increased risk of seizures within the first 48 h after radiosurgery, especially when treating a large lesion in eloquent cortex. Posttreatment seizures are often due to subtherapeutic levels of anticonvulsants in patients who are on these agents. Treatment consists of measuring serum anticonvulsant levels and providing additional medication when needed. At Stanford we regularly augment standard anticonvulsant doses to achieve a short-lived 'toxic' level in patients at high risk for posttreatment fits, thereby virtually preventing all seizures during the immediate posttreatment period.

Miscellaneous: Pin Site Pain, Headaches and Fever

The rigid skeletal fixation provided by a stereotactic frame is not suprisingly the most uncomfortable part of treatment (this situation, in part, has provided the impetus for developing a frameless stereotactic system [11]). The short duration of pain/headache during and throughout frame placement is typical, and generally not considered an adverse event. However, a few patients encounter pain at their pin sites for several days following removal of the stereotactic frame, because of small subcutaneous or subgaleal hematomas or irritation of superficial scalp nerves. Headaches may also be related to acute cerebral edema, as some authors have proposed [9]. Treatment consists of oral analgesics when needed. However, with operator experience, musculoskeletal pain can be significantly minimized by altering frame position so as to avoid the placement of pins in the temporalis muscle or adjacent to neural foramen, such as the superior orbital groove.

Kjellberg et al. [10] reported several patients with markedly elevated temperature following treatment of diencephalic AVMs with proton therapy, a phenomenon we have observed in 1 of our own patients at Stanford (maximum temperature: 106 °C). Acute edema within the hypothalamus seems likely to be the cause of such temperature dysfunction.

Early Delayed Sequelae

Hydrocephalus

Hydrocephalus occurring soon after treatment is usually related to the natural history of the patients' disease, particularly for tumors within or adjacent to the ventricular system, or from intraventricular hemorrhage from vascular lesions or tumors. Treatment is discussed below under late complications.

Alopecia

Though frequent in whole-brain radiation, alopecia is seldom a problem after radiosurgery. Loeffler et al. [7] reported 1 patient who developed alopecia

Table 1. Radiation necrosis following stereotactic radiosurgery for tumors

Group (first author)	Patients in series, n	Patients with necrosis		Equipment
		n	%	
Adler [13]	33	6	18	LINAC
Loeffler [7][1]	44	2	4.5	LINAC
Nedzi [14]	60	2	3	LINAC
McKenzie [9]	42	2	5	LINAC
Laing [12]	22	5	22	LINAC

[1] Tumors and AVMs.

6 weeks after treatment of a superficial AVM of the left parietal lobe. The involved scalp received approximately 400 cGy, and hair returned within 3 months. Laing et al. [12] treated 22 recurrent glioma patients with fractionated LINAC radiosurgery (range 30 Gy over 6 fractions to 50 Gy over 10 fractions), and noted small areas of alopecia while treating tumors close to the skull vault. At Stanford we have occasionally witnessed temporary alopecia in our patients with larger superficial lesions.

Late Delayed Complications

Radiation Necrosis and Edema

Radiation necrosis and edema remain the most debilitating of the late complications caused by stereotactic radiosurgery. Histologic changes in the affected brain consist of neuronal death, gliosis, and both endothelial proliferation and hyalinization. Adler et al. [13] reported that 6 of 33 patients (18%) treated with LINAC radiosurgery (mean dose 25 Gy, range 16–35) for metastatic tumors developed radiation-induced edema. All patients improved with oral steroids. The rate of necrosis following radiosurgery in other tumor and AVM series is shown in tables 1 and 2.

Nedzi et al. [14] retrospectively evaluated the variables associated with radiation necrosis and edema following radiosurgical treatment of 64 recurrent or inoperable intracranial tumors (60 patients); median follow-up was 8 months (range 2–43). The variables associated with significantly more toxicity are shown in table 3. Steiner et al. [15] reported more frequent radiation injury at higher doses, suggesting a possible threshold of 20 Gy when using larger (8 or 14 mm) gamma knife collimotors. Meanwhile, Flickinger [16] noted a

Table 2. Radiation necrosis following stereotactic radiosurgery for AVM

Group (first author)	Patients in series, n	Patients with necrosis		Equipment
		n	%	
Sutcliffe [35]	160	6	4	LINAC
Steiner [36]	300	7	2.3	Gamma knife
Steinberg [17]	86	17	20	Heavy particle
McKenzie [9]	70	3	4	LINAC

Table 3. Variables associated with increased risk radiation necrosis

Variable	p value
Tumor dose inhomogeneity	<0.00001
Maximum tumor dose	<0.00002
Number of isocenter	0.00002
Maximum normal tissue dose	0.00005
Tumor volume	0.001

Variables not associated with toxicity were mean tumor dose, number of treatment arcs, total degree of arc, tumor location, previous radiotherapy, tumor geometry, pretreatment performance status, collimator size, and age of patient.

similar threshold, which formed the basis for his integrated logistic formula. For AVMs, Steinberg et al. [17] noted that clinical complications were more frequent for doses > 18.5 Gy and volumes > 13 cm^3.

While radiation necrosis and edema often cause neurologic deterioration, tumor patients frequently suffer clinical deterioration as part of the natural progression of their disease. However, the MR and CT appearance of tumor progression (especially when necrotic) can be indistinguishable from radiation injury, both manifesting as contrast-enhancing lesions surrounded by significant edema. Consequently, it is often difficult to distinguish between radiation necrosis and tumor growth. Furthermore, even histopathology studies can be ambiguous. Biopsies taken from tumors treated with stereotactic radiosurgery often show regions of necrosis interspersed with live (but perhaps nonproliferative) tumor cells [18]. PET/SPECT scans can be helpful in distinguishing necrosis from tumor, but are frequently equivocal or falsely positive/negative.

The current mainstay of therapy for the late edema which occurs with radiation necrosis is corticosteroids; the course of symptoms and steroid treatment are typically quite protracted, lasting as long or longer than 1 year before resolving. In severe cases of necrosis, surgical resection can ameliorate mass effect and significantly improve some patients' clinical status.

Given the appreciable morbidity and protracted course of radiation necrosis, considerable effort has been directed at minimizing its incidence by optimizing treatment dose and restricting treatment volume to the targeted lesion as best as possible. Multiple retrospective studies have helped to refine treatment doses for most types of CNS tumors and vascular malformations. Meanwhile, new generations of radiosurgical technology, using either mini-multileaf collimators and more recently, robotic delivery systems without a discrete isocenter [11], allow for greater dose homogeneity and sharper dose fall-off outside the target. In addition, new pharmacologic treatments promise to yield additional therapies; Buatti et al. [19] reported in an animal model that lazaroids protect the normal brain from radiation injury produced by stereotactic radiosurgery.

Cranial Nerve Palsies

Cranial neuropathies are the most common adverse sequelae encountered with radiosurgery of skull base lesions. Furthermore, different cranial nerves have varying sensitivities to radiation, with motor nerves being more 'radioresistant' than sensory nerves. The optic nerve is the most sensitive of the cranial nerves [20, 21], followed by the cochlear [22–24] and the trigeminal nerves [22–24]. Studies have shown that the length of the cranial nerve radiated is a more important variable than the volume of tumor radiated when predicting the risk of postreatment cranial nerve dysfunction [25].

The exact tolerance of optic nerves and chiasm is unknown; threshold doses to this area have been arrived at empirically. From their experience, Backlund et al. [26] concluded that the tolerance of any portion of the optic nerve is approximately 10 Gy and planned treatment accordingly. Kondziolka et al. [20] of the University of Pittsburgh have empirically chosen to limit the dose to the optic chiasm to 8 Gy. Based on results from conventional fractionated radiotherapy, Loeffler et al. [7] also concluded that the tolerance of the optic system to a single fraction is approximately 10 Gy. Two patients developed a radiation-induced optic neuropathy following radiosurgery at Stanford, 1 of whom had a treatment dose as low as 8 Gy. In contrast, 1 patient treated at Stanford with an optic nerve sheath meningioma, retains vision, and even had improvement in her visual field and acuity, 5 years after treatment of her optic nerve with 25 Gy.

Trigeminal neuropathy is a complication that occurs most frequently with treatment of acoustic schwannoma. Noren et al. [27] reported that 18% of

110 patients with acoustic schwannomas treated with the gamma knife developed some degree of loss of facial sensation; symptoms correlated with maximum tumor doses of >30 Gy, while no patient treated with <27 Gy developed this complication. Flickinger et al. [28] reported a 37% incidence of trigeminal neuropathy 1 year following gamma knife treatment. The phenomenon of cranial nerve injury has also served as a basis for utilizing radiosurgery to treat functional disorders, such as trigeminal neuralgia; the early Stockholm experience revealed that radiosurgery with a dose of 180 Gy or higher produced small well-demarcated areas of necrosis [29, 30]. Although the trigeminal nerve is relatively prone to radiation injury at the root entry zone during the treatment of acoustic schwannomas, unexplainably the three divisions of this nerve seem quite impervious to much larger doses (>30 Gy) when treating lesions of the cavernous sinus region.

Facial nerve dysfunction is another not infrequent problem following radiosurgical treatment of acoustic schwannomas. In the above series by Noren et al. [27] and Flickinger et al. [28] of acoustic schwannoma patients, there was a 15 and 33% incidence of facial neuropathy. The usually transient disfigurement that results from the condition is particularly annoying to most patients.

The cochlear nerve is necessarily heavily irradiated when treating acoustic schwannomas although the vestibular nerve is in fact the typical nerve of origin for this unsuitably named lesion. A large proportion of such patients, particularly those with neurofibromatosis type II, have no useful hearing when they present. In others, however, useful hearing is present and an important goal of radiosurgery is to preserve this function. Hirsch and Noren [31] report on treating 126 patients, noting a 54% incidence of a unilateral deterioration in hearing and a 22% incidence of deafness. Kondziolka et al. [32] report that 23% of the 161 patients in their series had useful hearing prior to treatment, and the 2-year actuarial rate of *useful* hearing preservation in this group was $34.4 \pm 6.6\%$, while the 2-year actuarial rate of *some* hearing preservation was $71.0 \pm 4.4\%$. No cases of hearing loss were detected at any time beyond 22 months after radiosurgery. These results of hearing preservation are best interpreted in light of the natural history of acoustic schwannomas, which almost inevitably involves the gradual loss of hearing function.

The course of cranial nerve dysfunction following radiosurgery is variable. The vast majority of patients have partial injury which either improves appreciably or returns to normal with time (typically 1–2 years). Others, particularly the rare patient with complete facial palsies, have little or no improvement. Treatment with steroids has been of marginal benefit in our experience. Over the past decade there has been a gradual lowering of the dose used to treat acoustic neuroma, which has resulted in fewer cranial nerve complications without affecting, to date, tumor control. Preliminary experience suggests that complication rates, and especially hearing loss, can be decreased even further by utilizing some measure of treatment fractionation.

Transient Enlargement of Lesions

Radionecrosis usually results in either shrinkage or stabilization in the treated size of tumor or vascular malformation. However, in rare situations, a transient increase in lesion size has been observed. In one series of 55 skull base meningiomas treated with LINAC radiosurgery, one sphenoid wing meningioma was significantly larger on 3-month follow-up imaging, but decreased to less than initial treatment size at 9-month follow-up [6]. The same phenomenon has been antidotely observed both at Stanford and elsewhere in the treatment of some acoustic neuromas. Again, the mechanism for this phenomenon is believed to be intratumoral edema and is best treated with glucocorticoids. Nedzi et al. [14] describes 3 of 60 patients (5%) who required a decompression craniotomy following stereotactic radiosurgery, presumably for lesion enlargement. In most patients (especially with malignancies) lesion enlargement following radiosurgery more likely represents a failure of treatment. Inadequate radiosurgical dosing or a 'radioresistant' lesion are the most likely explanation when treatment fails. Again PET and SPECT scans can prove useful in distinguishing between transient tumor edema/necrosis and growth.

Hydrocephalus

Late hydrocephalus following stereotactic radiosurgery can occur for many reasons such as edema at the treatment site, tumor progression, hemorrhage within a tumor or vascular malformation, or most commonly scarring of the meninges. Nedzi et al. [14] reported that 3 of 60 patients (5%) in their series required shunting. Meanwhile, Thomsen et al. [33] describe a case of hydrocephalus developing 9 months after gamma knife treatment for an acoustic neuroma. Kondziolka et al. [32] reported that 4 of 161 patients treated with a gamma unit for acoustic neuromas developed hydrocephalus (median 7.5 months after treatment) requiring shunting. The presentation of hydrocephalus may be chronic (dementia, urinary incontinence, gait apraxia), or acute (headache, vomiting, altered mental status), with the latter most probable in the setting of hemorrhage from a nonobliterated AVM. Treatment consists of either transient CSF diversion or placement of a ventriculoperitoneal shunt.

Seizures

Late seizures, as with those observed in the acute phase, are typically part of the natural presentation of a disease. Although it has not been reported, de novo epilepsy could develop in an area of radiation injury with necrosis and edema serving as seizure foci. Instead, several centers in Europe are actually investigating the utility of radiosurgical ablation in destroying small nonvisible epileptiform foci. Long-term anticonvulsants, and sometimes steroid therapy, are the treatment of choice.

Hormonal Abnormalities

Changes in the hormonal axis of a patient can occur with stereotactic radiosurgery of lesions within or adjacent to the pituitary gland or hypothalamus. However, many patients with sella tumors already have hypopituitary dysfunction prior to radiosurgery. Degerblad et al. [34] used radiosurgery to treat a diffusely hyperactive pituitary gland in 35 patients with Cushing's disease; only 12 patients (32%) developed pituitary insufficiency following radiosurgery (with gonadotropin, thyrotropin or corticotropin failure). Unlike conventional pituitary radiation therapy, the precision of targeting with radiosurgery permits a treatment to be localized to a small hormonally active microadenoma if it can be visualized on imaging studies. Nevertheless, some measure of dose is delivered to normal pituitary which risks pituitary deficiency over the long term. With advances in radiosurgical targeting it should be possible to further minimize the likelihood of panhypopituitarism. When hormonal deficiency does occur, treatment consists of appropriate supplementation with exogenous hormones.

In summary: Despite the great strides made in stereotactic radiosurgery over the last severel decades, it is not complication-free. While the list of potential sequelae is substantial, few result in permanent disability and the vast majority of patients have no long-term adverse effects. Meanwhile, many of the reported 'complications' after radiosurgery appear to represent the consequences of the disease progression and not side effects from treatment. Future advances in radiosurgical technology and treatment planning promise to further reduce complications.

References

1   Leksell L: The stereotactic method and radiosurgery of the brain. Acta Chir Scand 1951;102: 316–319.
2   Sheline GE, Wara WM, Smith V: Therapeutic irradiation and brain injury. Int J Radiat Oncol Biol Phys 1980;6:1215–1228.
3   Kondziolka D, Somaza S, Comey C et al: Radiosurgery and fractionated radiation therapy: Comparison of different techniques in an in vivo rat glioma model. J Neurosurg 1996;84:1033–1038.
4   Nakata H, Yoshimine T, Murasawa A et al: Early blood-brain barrier disruption after high-dose single-fraction irradiation in rats. Acta Neurochir (Wien) 1995;136:82–87.
5   Inoue HK, Kohga H, Hirato M et al: Neurobiologic effects of radiosurgery: Histologic, immunohistochemical and electron-microscopic studies of a rat model. Stereotact Funct Neurosurg 1994;63: 280–285.

6   Chang SD, Adler JR: Treatment of cranial base meningiomas with LINAC radiosurgery. Neuro-surgery 1997;41:1019–1027.

7   Loeffler JS, Siddon RL, Wen PY et al: Stereotactic radiosurgery of the brain using a standard linear accelerator: A study of early and late effects. Radiother Oncol 1990;17:311–321.

8   Bodis S, Alexander ER, Kooy H et al: The prevention of radiosurgery-induced nausea and vomiting by ondansetron: Evidence of a direct effect on the central nervous system chemoreceptor trigger zone. Surg Neurol 1994;42:249–252.

9   McKenzie MR, Souhami L, Caron JL et al: Early and late complications following dynamic stereotactic radiosurgery and fractionated stereotactic radiotherapy. Can J Neurol Sci 1993;20:279–285.

10   Kjellberg RN, Davis KR, Lyons S et al: Bragg peak proton beam therapy for arteriovenous malforma-tion of the brain. Clin Neurosurg 1983;31:248–290.

11   Adler JR, Cox RS: Preliminary clinical experience with the Cyberknife: Image-guided stereotactic radiosurgery; in Kondziolka D (eds): Radiosurgery 1995. Basel, Karger, 1996, pp 316–326.

12   Laing RW, Warrington AP, Graham J et al: Efficacy and toxicity of fractionated stereotactic radiotherapy in the treatment of recurrent gliomas (phase I/II study). Radiother Oncol 1993;27:22–29.

13   Adler JR, Cox RS, Kaplan I et al: Stereotactic radiosurgical treatment of brain metastasis. J Neuro-surg 1992;76:444–449.

14   Nedzi LA, Kooy H, Alexander ED et al: Variables associated with the development of complications from radiosurgery of intracranial tumors. Int J Radiat Oncol Biol Phys 1991;21:591–599.

15   Steiner L, Greitz T, Backlund EO et al: Radiosurgery in arteriovenous malformations of the brain; in Szikla G (ed): Stereotactic Cerebral Irradiation. Amsterdam, Elsevier/North-Holland Biomedical Press, 1979, pp 257–269.

16   Flickinger JC: An integrated logistic formula for prediction of complications from radiosurgery. Int J Radiat Oncol Biol Phys 1989;17:879–885.

17   Steinberg GK, Fabrikant JI, Marks MP et al: Stereotactic heavy-charged-particle Bragg-peak radiation for intracranial arteriovenous malformations [see comments]. N Engl J Med 1990;323:96–101.

18   Harris OA, Adler JA Jr: Analysis of the proliferative potential of residual tumor after radiosurgery for intraparenchymal brain metastasis. J Neurosurg 1996;85:667–671.

19   Buatti JM, Friedman WA, Theele DP et al: The lazaroid U74389G protects normal brain from stereotactic radiosurgery-induced radiation injury. Int J Radiat Oncol Biol Phys 1996;34:591–597.

20   Kondziolka D, Lunsford LD, Coffey RJ et al: Stereotactic radiosurgery of meningiomas. J Neurosurg 1991;74:552–559.

21   Kondziolka D, Lunsford LD: Radiosurgery of meningiomas. Neurosurg Clin North Am 1992;3:219–230.

22   Linskey ME, Lunsford LD, Flickinger JC: Radiosurgery for acoustic neurinomas: Early experience. Neurosurgery 1990;26:736–745.

23   Linskey ME, Lunsford LD, Flickinger JC: Neuroimaging of acoustic nerve sheath tumors after stereotaxic radiosurgery. AJNR Am J Neuroradiol 1991;12:1165–1175.

24   Linskey M, Lunsford L, Flickinger J: Tumor control after stereotactic radiosurgery in neurofibro-matosis patients with bilateral acoustic tumors. Neurosurgery 1992;31:829–839.

25   Linskey ME, Flickinger JC, Lunsford LD: Cranial nerve length predicts the risk of delayed facial and trigeminal neuropathies after acoustic tumor stereotactic radiosurgery. Int J Radiat Oncol Biol Phys 1993;25:227–233.

26   Backlund EO, Bergstrand G, Hierton-Laurell U et al: Tumor changes after single dose irradiation by stereotactic radiosurgery in 'nonactive' pituitary adenomas and prolactinomas; in Szikla G (ed): Stereotactic Cerebral Irradiation. Amsterdam, Elsevier/North-Holland Biomedical Press, 1979, pp 199–206.

27   Noren G, Arndt J, Hinmarsh T: Stereotactic radiosurgical treatment of acoustic neurinomas; in Lunsford LD (ed): Modern Stereotactic Neurosurgery. Boston, Nijhoff, 1988, pp 481–489.

28   Flickinger JC, Lunsford LD, Coffey RJ et al: Radiosurgery of acoustic neurinomas. Cancer 1991;67:345–353.

29 Leksell L: Cerebral radiosurgery. I. Gammathalanotomy in two cases of intractable pain. Acta Chir Scand 1968;134:585–595.

30 Leksell L, Herner T, Leksell D et al: Visualisation of stereotactic radiolesions by nuclear magnetic resonance. J Neurol Neurosurg Psychiatry 1985;48:19–20.

31 Hirsch A, Noren G: Audiological findings after stereotactic radiosurgery in acoustic neurinomas. Acta Otolaryngol (Stockh) 1988;106:244–251.

32 Kondziolka D, Lunsford L, Linskey M et al: Skull base radiosurgery; in Alexander EI, Loeffler J, Lunsford L (eds): Stereotactic Radiosurgery. New York, McGraw-Hill, 1993, pp 175–188.

33 Thomsen J, Tos M, Borgesen SE: Gamma knife: Hydrocephalus as a complication of stereotactic radiosurgical treatment of an acoustic neuroma. Am J Otol 1990;11:330–333.

34 Degerblad M, Rahn T, Bergstrand G et al: Long-term results of stereotactic radiosurgery to the pituitary gland in Cushing's disease. Acta Endocrinol (Copenh) 1986;112:310–314.

35 Sutcliffe JC, Forster DM, Walton L et al: Untoward clinical effects after stereotactic radiosurgery for intracranial arteriovenous malformations. Br J Neurosurg 1992;6:177–185.

36 Steiner L: Stereotactic radiosurgery with the cobalt-60 gamma unit in the surgical treatment of intracranial tumors and arteriovenous malformations; in Schmidek HH, Sweet WH (eds): Operative Neurosurgical Techniques – Indications, Methods, and Results. Philadelphia, Saunders, 1988, pp 515–529.

John R. Adler, MD, Department of Neurosurgery, Stanford Medical Center,
300 Pasteur Drive, Stanford CA 94305 (USA)
Tel. +1 650 723 5573, Fax +1 650 723 7813

Author Index

Subject Index

Eye, radiation injury (continued)
conjunctiva injection 130
dry-eye syndrome 23, 24, 132, 133, 135
eyelids
clinical syndromes 22, 127, 129
treatment 127
fornix contraction, surgical management
131, 132
lacrimal duct injury
clinical syndromes 132, 133
overview 22, 132
treatment 133, 135
optic nerve injury
clinical presentation 139
dose response 28, 30, 160
management 30, 139
neuropathy types 27, 28
sensitization by chemotherapy 29
orbit injury
clinical syndromes 141, 142
treatment 142
prevention 21, 31, 32
retinopathy
dose response 26
features 25, 26, 136–138
management 27, 138
sclera injury 130, 132

Fatigue, radiation side effect and
mechanisms 7
Fistula, radiation injury and management
57, 58
5-Fluorouracil
leucovorin combination therapy 115, 116
radiosensitization for gastrointestinal
tract cancer treatment
chemoradiation as accelerated
treatment
anal cancer 114, 115
esophageal cancer 114
head and neck cancer 113, 114
overview 113
circadian timing of administration
116, 117
metastatic colorectal cancer treatment
112
overview 110

protracted venous infusion of drug
110–112
treatment planning 117
Fornix contraction, surgical management
131, 132

Granulocyte colony-stimulating factor,
prophylaxis of radiation injury 10
Granulocyte-macrophage colony-
stimulating factor, prophylaxis of
radiation injury 10

Heart, radiation injury
conducting abnormality 83
coronary artery disease
prevention 81, 82
risk factors 79–81
overview 71, 72
pericardial injury
clinical manifestations 75, 76, 78, 79
dose response 73, 74
Hodgkin's disease patients 73–75
prevention 74, 75
treatment 79
pleural effusion 83
tachyardia 83
valve defects 82, 83
Hemorrhagic cystitis
clinical features 120, 121
prevention 121
treatment 121–123
Hodgkin's disease
chemotherapy 86, 88, 89, 92, 93, 95
laparotomy in staging and
recommendations 86–88, 94
mortality 85
radiation therapy
combination with chemotherapy
92, 93
guidelines 85, 86, 90–92, 95
pericardial radiation injury and
prevention 73–75
recurrent disease 93, 94
Hydrocephalus, radiosurgery complications
157, 162
Hyperbaric oxygen
children, therapy 105

claustrophobia of patients 101
diseases for therapy 98, 101–105
fibroblast response 99
mechanism of action 99
osteoradionecrosis treatment 54, 55,
    102, 103
overview 98
toxicity and side effects 100
vasoconstriction 99
white cell killing enhancement 99

Incontinence, radiation injury 123, 124

Kidney, radiation tolerance 4

Lacrimal duct injury
    clinical syndromes 132, 133
    overview 22, 132
    treatment 133, 135
Late response
    radiation injury 1, 8, 10, 11
    radiosurgery 158–163
γ-Linolenic acid, prophylaxis of radiation
    injury 13–16
Lung, radiation injury
    acinus loss 65, 66
    conformal therapy in prevention 67, 68
    local control and prognosis 66, 67
    pneumonitis 6, 64, 68
    pulmonary fibrosis 64, 65
    reactive cell proliferation 65
    tolerance 63, 64
    transforming growth factor-β role in
        injury 64, 68

Magnetic resonance imaging
    conformal radiotherapy planning 67, 68
    edema 159
Mouth, radiation injury
    candidiasis 41
    dental caries 38, 39
    dental treatment planning 46–48
    mucositis 34, 35, 50
    nutritional management 38
    salivary function 37, 51
    soft tissue necrosis 45, 46
    taste loss 35, 36

Mucositis, features and management
    34, 35, 50

Nausea, radiosurgery complications 156

Optic nerve, radiation injury
    clinical presentation 139
    dose response 28, 30, 160
    management 30, 139
    neuropathy types 27, 28
    sensitization by chemotherapy 29
Orbit, radiation injury
    clinical syndromes 141, 142
    treatment 142
Osteoradionecrosis, head and neck
    diagnosis 53, 54
    incidence 42
    pathophysiology 52
    reconstructive surgery 55, 56
    recovery 41
    risk factors 44, 45, 52
    treatment 41, 42, 45, 54, 55, 102, 103

Penicillamine, prophylaxis of radiation
    injury 11
Pentoxyfylline
    palliative treatment 17
    prophylaxis of radiation injury 12
Pericardial injury
    clinical manifestations 75, 76, 78, 79
    Hodgkin disease patients 73–75
    prevention 74, 75
    radiation dose response 73, 74
    treatment 79
Pituitary hormones, radiosurgery
    complications 163
Pleural effusion, radiation injury 83
Pneumonitis, see Lung, radiation injury
Pulmonary fibrosis, see Lung, radiation
    injury

Radiosurgery
    acute complications
        edema 156
        fever 157
        nausea 156
        neurologic deterioration 156